# INTERMITTENT FASTING FOR WOMEN OVER 50

THE NEW APPROACH FOR SENIOR WOMEN TO DELAY AGING WHILE LOSING WEIGHT & PROMOTE LONGEVITY THROUGH METABOLIC AUTOPHAGY

KATE MCCARTHY

© **Copyright 2021—All rights reserved.**

It is not legal to reproduce, duplicate, or transmit any part of this document in either electronic means or in printed format. Recording of this publication is strictly prohibited and any storage of this document is not allowed unless with written permission from the publisher except for the use of brief quotations in a book review.

DOWNLOAD YOUR FREE CHEAT SHEET

*(Don't start fasting before you've consulted this cheat sheet...)*

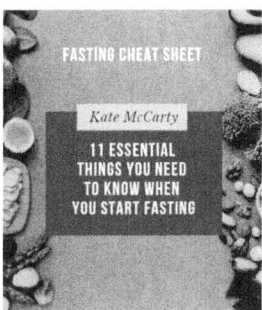

This cheat sheet includes:

- 11 things to know and to do while you are fasting.
- Why you need to know those things to start successfully.
- These things will make the process easier and more enjoyable.

The last thing I want is that the fasting process will be uncomfortable.

To receive your fasting cheat sheet, scan this QR code:

# CONTENTS

*Introduction*     9

1. DEFINITION OF INTERMITTENT FASTING     15
   Types of Intermittent Fasting     16
   The Stages of Intermittent Fasting     17
   The Science Behind Intermittent Fasting     20
   What Is Autophagy?     21
   Nine Advantages of Intermittent Fasting     24

2. YOUR BODY CHANGES IN UNEXPECTED WAYS AFTER 50     31
   Changes     32

3. CHOOSING THE RIGHT TYPE OF FASTING     46
   1. What Is 16/8 Intermittent Fasting?     47
   2. What Is 5:2 Intermittent Fasting?     50
   3. What Is Eat Stop Eat Intermittent Fasting?     53
   4. What Is Alternate-Day Fasting?     59
   5. What Is 12:12 Intermittent Fasting?     62

4. THE DOS AND DON'TS OF INTERMITTENT FASTING     65
   The Dos     65
   The Don'ts     72

5. EMBRACING THE LIFESTYLE     82
   1. Intermittent Fasting Isn't a Fad Diet; It's a Healthy Way of Life     82
   2. Listen to Your Body When It Comes to Deciding What To Eat     83
   3. It Simplifies Your Life     84

| | |
|---|---|
| 4. After a Year Or So, You Might Expect Your Results To Slow Down | 84 |
| 5. Fast Fat Reduction Is Achieved By Combining Intermittent Fasting with High-Intensity Interval Training | 85 |
| 6. Intermittent Fasting Can Help You Focus, Be More Productive, And Be More Disciplined | 85 |
| 7. Fasting on a Regular Basis Might Affect Your Discipline, Focus, And Productivity | 86 |
| 8. Intermittent Fasting May Wreak Havoc on Your Diet | 87 |
| 9. Intermittent Fasting Has Been Linked to Muscle Loss Or Increase | 87 |
| 10. Because It Allows You to Consume Fewer Calories, Intermittent Fasting Is Effective. | 88 |
| 11. Allowing Yourself to Fast Intermittently Should Not Keep You From Living Your Life | 89 |
| Let's Get Started: The Steps | 90 |
| Conclusion | 98 |
| 6. COMBINE INTERMITTENT FASTING WITH HEALTHY HABITS | 99 |
| Precontemplation | 100 |
| Contemplation: "I'm thinking about it." | 100 |
| Preparation: "I've made up my mind to do something." | 101 |
| Acton: "I've begun to make changes." | 101 |
| Maintenance: "I've adopted a new routine." | 102 |
| Is It Better to Develop Healthy Habits Alone Or with the Help of a Support Group? | 103 |
| What Are the Advantages of Having a Healthy Eating Support System? | 103 |
| Is It True that Having a Support System Can Help You Achieve Your Weight-Loss Goals? | 104 |
| What Small, Healthy Improvements Can I Make at Home Today? | 105 |
| Healthy Habits | 108 |

7. BREAKFAST RECIPES ... 118
   1. Sweet Potatoes with Egg Scramble ... 119
   2. Turmeric Tofu Scrambles ... 120
   3. Avocado Ricotta Power Toast ... 121
   4. Almond Apple Spice Muffins ... 122
   5. Bowl of Roasted Veggies and Savory Oats ... 123
   6. Spinach and Bacon Mini Quiches ... 125
   7. Buddha Bowl ... 126
   8. Berry Matcha Smoothie ... 128
   9. Feta-Filled Tomato-Topped Oldie Omelette ... 129
   10. Carrot Breakfast Salad ... 130
   11. Delicious Turkey Wrap ... 131
   12. Bacon and Chicken Garlic Wrap ... 132
   13. Pumpkin Pancakes ... 133
   14. Cheddar Ham Frittata ... 134
   15. Orange Rasp French Toast ... 135
   16. Cinnamon Stevia Oatmeal ... 136

8. LUNCH RECIPES ... 138
   1. Chicken Farro Bowl ... 138
   2. Shrimp Fried Rice ... 141
   3. Grass-Fed Burgers ... 142
   4. Shrimp And Avocado Salad ... 144
   5. Buffalo Chicken Chopped Salad ... 145
   6. Salmon Sesame Pak Choi ... 147
   7. Grilled Chicken Salad ... 148
   8. Steak Fajita Power Bowl ... 150
   9. Mango Chili Chicken Stir-Fry ... 151
   10. Turkey with Capers, Tomatoes, and Green Beans ... 153
   11. Thai Fish Curry ... 154
   12. Fried Tofu with Tender Spring Greens ... 155
   13. Satisfying Turkey Lettuce Wraps ... 156

9. DINNER RECIPES — 158
  1. Turkey Tacos — 158
  2. Spaghetti Bolognese — 159
  3. Chicken with Fried Cauliflower Rice — 161
  4. Sheet-Pan Steak — 163
  5. Zoodles with Keto Alfredo Sauce — 164
  6. Pork Tenderloin with Butternut Squash and Brussels Sprouts — 166
  7. Beef and Carrot Stew — 168

*Conclusion* — 171
*References* — 177

# INTRODUCTION

> "Take away food from a sick man's stomach and you have begun, not to starve the sick man, but the disease."
>
> — E.H. DEWEY, MD

Many of us seek ways to heal and, ideally, reverse the harm we have done to our bodies by living in this age of perpetual stress, worry, and rising levels of chronic illness. While the World Health Organization designated malnutrition, or famine, as the most important global health issue twenty years ago, we now face the polar opposite. Overnutrition, which leads to obesity, has emerged as the world's most pressing health issue, especially in developing countries. Obesity is a substantial risk factor for a variety of chronic conditions, including heart disease, diabetes, and high blood pressure. As a result of this shift in global health dynamics, several trendy diets and self-proclaimed experts have emerged, promising you immediate, dramatic, and long-term weight loss with no scientific evidence or social proof to back up their claims. Unfortunately, trendy diets typically cause more harm than good in the long run. While you may lose weight, you never know what long-term damage may be done to your body because these new and experimental diets and eating programs are generally the unscientific brainchild of nonprofessionals. On the other hand, even if these trendy diets work, they will just help you lose weight and provide no other health benefits. Fasting differs in this regard.

Fasting has thousands of years of scientific and sociological proof behind it as an age-old practice. The celebration of Ramadan, a Muslim fasting time, is perhaps one of the most well-known religious and spiritual connections to fasting. Participants in the Ramadan fast have demonstrated a better immunological response during this time, which shows that fasting has a favorable effect on the body. Fasting is a way of life that can help you lose weight healthily while also providing a variety of other health benefits. Although fasting dates back to ancient times, it has recently acquired appeal as a method of weight loss and health improvement. This unexpected rise in public interest has also resulted in a lot of misinformation, so it's critical to define its origins and purposes, as well as the scientific basis for how fasting works, in order to fully understand and use it to its full potential. Fortunately, fasting is the research community's sweetheart since it routinely produces demonstrable outcomes in clinical settings, so you'll have plenty of facts and knowledge to work with when deciding whether or not fasting is good for you.

Fasting is likely something you are already familiar with, but for the sake of clarity, I'd like to describe the notion for you here. Fasting is defined as the voluntary restriction of food consumption to specific times. Fasting is not the same as starving, which is a case in which you are being forced to go without food and that causes harm to your body. Fasting, on the other hand, is the polar opposite. Fasting as part of a healthy lifestyle can help you lose weight while also triggering and speeding up natural processes in your body that promote better overall physical, mental, and emotional health. Our bodies are not designed to be constantly fed, and when we deny ourselves food, our bodies respond positively. Hormones are released into the bloodstream to regulate our appetite, maintain our glucose levels, boost our metabolic response, and even influence our nervous system.

I believe it's equally vital for me to tell you how I came to learn about water fasting and how it has helped me. In my early twenties, I began to develop insulin resistance. It affected my weight, raised my diabetes risk, and I felt compelled to take the meds that the physicians gave at such a young age. My insulin sensitivity did not increase enough to return me to the life I had before, despite pharmaceutical and dietary therapies. This had a profound emotional impact on me, and I felt as if my youth was being robbed from me. When I turned thirty, I was inspired to make healthier lifestyle choices and began investigating holistic and alternative methods. This is when I first learned about intermittent fasting and, more crucially, water fasting. I began combining both into my daily routine, as well as mindfulness, meditation, and proper dietary selections. I was able to lose seventy-five pounds over time. My insulin sensitivity had improved to the point that my physicians said I could stop taking my meds.

Years later, and still in good health, I've compiled all of my findings and personal practices into two books: Water Fasting and One Meal a Day Intermittent Fasting. I wrote these books with a lot of love and care for others, hoping that by sharing this wisdom, others may be able to transform their lives and reap the benefits of such easy activities.

You probably bought this book because you have physical problems that need to be addressed—wanting to lose excess weight, chronic sickness, or simply a desire to improve your longevity and cognitive functioning. My wish for you is that by the end of this book, you will have the knowledge and skills necessary to apply intermittent fasting as a lifestyle solution to these health problems, and that you will feel confident in your ability to do so.

This book is intended to be a comprehensive reference for you as you embark on your intermittent fasting adventure. It will provide you with all of the necessary tools and answer any questions you may have regarding intermittent fasting. Your intermittent fasting journey is about to begin. When we grow up, we go through a bit of pain as our bodies adjust to their growth spurts and mental achievements. When we work out, we feel the burn at first, only to see the wonderful results we get afterward. Everything comes with a bit of growing pain, you see, but the greener pastures beyond adversity mean so much more than the initial struggle.

## 1

## DEFINITION OF INTERMITTENT FASTING

A practice called intermittent fasting, at this time, is one of the world's most known health and fitness trends. It involves interchanging rotations of fasting and eating. Many studies indicate that this can bring about weight loss, better metabolic health, safeguard against disease, and perhaps aid you in living longer. This book describes what intermittent fasting is, and why you should care.

To understand what it is all about, intermittent fasting is an eating arrangement where you rotate between episodes of food intake and fasting. The focus is not on what kinds of food to eat, but rather on the time periods for food consumption. There are various intermittent fasting approaches, all of them are divided into a timeframe of weeks or days of consuming food phases and fasting phases. A lot of individuals by now fast on a daily basis, while slumbering. An individual can exercise intermittent fasting by missing breakfast, consuming their first meal at noon, and their last meal at 8 p.m. At this point they're officially fasting for sixteen hours daily, and containing their food intake to an eight-hour intake gap. This method is a common formula of fasting, called the 16/8 approach. Regardless of what you might think, intermittent fasting is a fairly stress-free process. A lot of people give feedback of feeling healthy and experiencing more vitality for the duration of a fast. Desire for food is generally not that problematic; nevertheless it can prove challenging at the start, as your body is getting acclimated to not taking food for prolonged episodes of time. Food is usually not acceptable all through the fasting session, however you can drink tea, water, coffee, and other drinks that do not contain calories. Other methods of fasting tolerate a bit of small-calorie diets for the period of the fasting session. Consumption of supplements is normally allowed, provided they have no calories.

## TYPES OF INTERMITTENT FASTING

Intermittent fasting has grown in popularity in the previous few years, and several different methods have appeared. Below are some of the most common ones:

- **16/8 Approach:** Fast for sixteen hours daily. For instance, only consuming food between noon and 8 p.m.
- **Eat Stop Eat:** Once to twice a week, don't eat

anything from supper one day, until supper the next day (a twenty-four-hour fast).

- **5:2 Diet:** Throughout two days of the week, consume only 500 to 600 calories.

Then there are many other distinctions.

## THE STAGES OF INTERMITTENT FASTING

**1. Fed State**

Your blood sugar levels will rise during this time, and you will secrete more insulin. Insulin is the hormone that transports sugar from the bloodstream into your cells. The amount of insulin released is determined by the composition of your meal, the amount of carbohydrates eaten, and your body's insulin sensitivity. Extra glucose (sugar) is stored as glycogen in the liver and muscles. Glycogen is your body's main source of stored carbohydrates, and it can be turned back into sugar as needed. Other hormones, like leptin and ghrelin, also fluctuate during this time. Ghrelin is a hunger-stimulating hormone, and its levels decrease after you eat. Meanwhile, after eating, the hormone leptin, which suppresses appetite, surges. It's worth noting that when food is consumed during a fast, the fed-fast cycle resets to the fed state. In addition, the size and substance of your meal has an impact on how long your body stays in a satiated state.

## 2. Early Fasting State

Your body enters an early fasting state three to four hours after you've eaten, which lasts for about eighteen hours after you eat. Your insulin and blood sugar levels begin to drop during this phase, causing your body to begin converting glycogen into glucose for energy. By the end of this phase, your body will have depleted its liver glycogen stores and will be looking for another source of energy. This speeds up lipolysis, a process in which fat cells' triglycerides are broken down into smaller molecules, which can be used as a source of alternative energy. Amino acids, which are the building blocks of proteins, are also converted into energy by your body. Many prevalent kinds of intermittent fasting, such as the 16/8 approach, alternate between being fed and fasting early.

## 3. Fasting State

The fasting period might last anywhere from eighteen hours to two days. Your liver's glycogen stores are depleted at this stage, and your body starts breaking down protein and fat stores for energy instead. Ketone bodies, a sort of substance formed when your body transforms fat into fuel, are produced as a result of this. This also leads your body to enter ketosis, a metabolic condition in which fat serves as your body's principal source of energy. The transition into ketosis, on the other hand, may not occur immediately when you enter the fasting state, but sometime later. The size and nature of your typical diet and last meal, as well as individual differences, influence how quickly you break your fast. Reduced appetite, weight loss, weariness, unpleasant or fruity-smelling breath, and high levels of ketone bodies in the blood, breath, or urine, are some of the most typical indications of ketosis.

Ketosis can also be achieved by other techniques, such as adhering to the ketogenic diet, which entails drastically reducing carbohydrate intake. Keep in mind that ketosis is not to be confused with ketoacidosis, which is a severe disease caused by your blood becoming overly acidic. Ketoacidosis, unlike ketosis, is caused by disease, infection, or poorly managed diabetes, and it necessitates rapid medical intervention. Also, notice that forms of intermittent fasting with shorter fasting windows of twelve to eighteen hours per day may not accomplish this state, as ketosis cannot be achieved with fasts of fewer than twenty-four hours unless you also follow an extremely low-carb diet.

## 4. Long-Term Fasting State

Your body enters the long-term fasting state after protracted durations of fasting, which usually happens forty-eight hours following meal intake. This is described as the "starvation condition" by some. The normal response of your body to long-term calorie restriction is known as "starvation mode" (and occasionally, "metabolic damage"). To maintain energy balance and avoid famine, the body responds to lower calorie intake by lowering calorie expenditure. Adaptive thermogenesis is the technical term for this natural physiological reaction. True hunger is virtually wholly irrelevant to most weight reduction talks, hence the term "starvation mode" is a misnomer. In today's food economy, where obesity is common, starvation mode is a useful physiological response, but it does more harm than good.

Insulin levels will continue to fall in the long-term fasting state, while beta-hydroxybutyrate (BHB), a form of ketone body, progressively grows. Your kidneys also continue to produce sugar through a process known as gluconeogenesis, which is the brain's primary source of fuel. At this moment, ketone bodies also provide energy to the brain. The breakdown of three important amino acids, branched-chain amino acids (BCAAs), also decreases to help the body conserve muscular tissue. Remember that long-term fasting is not recommended for the majority of individuals and should only be done under medical supervision.

## THE SCIENCE BEHIND INTERMITTENT FASTING

Understanding the science behind why intermittent fasting works will help you to feel confident and comfortable as you change your diet and lifestyle to accommodate this new regime. We will begin by answering the question of what autophagy is, before moving on to more specific aspects of this interesting cellular process in the body.

## WHAT IS AUTOPHAGY?

Autophagy is a process that occurs in humans, and it has been unknowingly occurring since the birth of humankind. Until recently, people began to use this process to achieve the desired positive results by changing their diet (such as intermittent fasting). We will look at this topic in-depth throughout this book, but here we will begin by looking at what exactly autophagy is.

Autophagy, as a word, can be broken up into two individual parts. Each of these parts on its own is a separate Greek word—the word auto means self, and the word phagy means the practice of eating. Putting these together gives you the practice of self-eating, which is essentially what autophagy is. This may sound a little intimidating. Still, it is a very natural process that our cells practice all the time without us being any the wiser. Autophagy is the body's way of cleaning itself out.

Essentially, the body has housekeepers that keep everything neat and tidy. Scientists who have been studying this for some time are now beginning to understand that there are ways to manipulate this process within your body to achieve things such as weight loss, improved health, reduction of disease symptoms, and so on. This is what we will spend the rest of the book looking at, but first, we will dive into the science of autophagy a little more.

The process of autophagy involves small "hunter" particles that go around your body, looking for cells or cell components that are old and damaged. The hunter particles then take these cell components apart, getting rid of the damaged parts and saving the useful parts to make new cells later. These hunter cells can also use useful leftover parts to create energy for the body.

Autophagy has been found to happen in all organisms that are multicellular, like animals and plants, in addition to humans. Although there is minimal research on these larger organisms and their effects on autophagy, there are more and more studies on humans and how dietary changes affect human autophagy.

The other function that autophagy serves is that it helps cells to carry out their death, when it is time for them to die. There are times when cells are programmed to die because of several different factors. Sometimes these cells need assistance in their death, and autophagy can help them with this or can help to clean up after their death. The human body is all about life and death. These processes are continually going on without our knowledge to keep us healthy and in good form.

As I mentioned, the autophagy process has been going on inside of us for many, many years, since the beginning of humankind. This process has been kept around inside our bodies because of the many benefits it can provide us. It is also essential for our bodies' health, as being able to get rid of waste and damaged parts that are no longer useful to us is essential to our health. If we could not get rid of damaged or broken cells, these damaged particles would build up and eventually make us sick. Our bodies are extremely efficient in everything that they do, and waste disposal is no different.

In more recent years, the study of autophagy has been focused more heavily on diet and disease research. These studies are still in their early stages, as it has been only slightly shy of sixty years since autophagy was first discovered. This process was discovered in a lab by testing what happened when small organisms went without food for some time. These organisms were observed very closely under a microscope. It was found that their cells had this process of waste disposal and energy creation that was later named autophagy.

More about autophagy and its relation to energy production is currently being studied. Autophagy can use old cell parts and recycle them to create new energy that the organism (like the human or animal) can use to do its regular functions like walking and breathing. Now, people are studying what happens when humans rely on this form of energy production instead of the energy they would get from ingesting food throughout the day. This is where autophagy and intermittent fasting come together. We will look at how they work together throughout the rest of this book as we delve deeply into intermittent fasting and autophagy and how they work together to allow for things like weight loss or disease prevention.

# NINE ADVANTAGES OF INTERMITTENT FASTING

Intermittent fasting is a food consumption practice where you rotate between episodes of intake of food and not taking food. A lot of different methods of intermittent fasting exist, such as the 16/8 and 5:2 approaches. A lot of research illustrates that it can have great gains for your physique and brain. Below are nine health gains of fasting:

## 1. Changes the Function of Hormones, Cells, and Genes

When you stop eating for some time, a couple of things will occur in your physique. Take for instance, your body modifies hormone levels to make deposited body fat more available and starts the important cellular patch-up processes. Below are some of the happenings that occur in your body during fasting:

- **Insulin points.** Blood levels of insulin go down significantly, which helps with burning fat.
- **Human development hormone levels.** The amount of human growth hormone in your blood may rise radically. Higher points of this hormone aid fat reduction and muscle development, and contain numerous other benefits.
- **Cellular patch-up.** The body makes important

cellular healing processes, such as eliminating unwanted material from cells.
- **Gene expression.** There are valuable modifications in some genes and molecules related to a long lifespan and strong defenses against illness.

## 2. Can Help You Lose Weight and Visceral Fat

A lot of people who attempt fasting are undertaking it to cut down on weight. Generally, fasting will make you consume less meals. Lest you pay off by eating greatly more in the course of the other diets, you'll end up losing weight.

Furthermore, intermittent fasting increases hormone production to help in shedding weight. Lesser insulin levels, upped HGH amounts, and enhanced quantities of norepinephrine will raise the disintegration of body fat. For this purpose, short-period fasting really adds to your digestion rate, helps to shed even more calories. In other terms, fasting works equally on both ends of the calorie balance. It increases your digestion rate and cuts the amount of food you consume. In accordance with a 2014 research review, intermittent fasting was able to shed weight of 3 to 8 percent in a duration of three to twenty-four weeks. This is a significant amount. In the research, partakers also shed 4 to 7 percent of their waistline circumference over weeks six to twenty-four, which indicates that they did shed lots of mass. Visceral fat is dangerous fat in the stomach cavity that causes illness. One 2011 assessment also indicates that fasting has fewer muscle shed effects than constant calorie limitation. Nevertheless, a 2020 randomized test looked at individuals who tracked the 16/8 process. In this method, you fast for sixteen hours per day and have an eight-hour gap to consume food. Individuals who fasted didn't shed meaningfully more weight than the individual who consumed three meals in a day. After trying a subgroup of the participants in-person, scientists also realized that the individuals who fasted did shed a substantial amount of thin mass. It encompassed lean muscle. Additional studies are required to find out the outcome of fasting on muscle shed. In consideration of all factors, well thought out intermittent fasting has the possibility to be an unbelievably great tool of losing weight.

## 3. Can Reduce Insulin Resistance, Lowering Your Risk for Type 2 Diabetes

Type 2 diabetes has turned into a very common diagnosis in recent years. Its key characteristics are high levels of blood sugar and insulin resistance. Fascinatingly, intermittent fasting's main advantage is insulin resistance and causes a remarkable decrease in blood sugar levels. In human research on fasting, fasting blood sugar contributed to a decrease of 3 to 6 percent in individuals with prediabetes. Fasting insulin dropped by 20 to 31 percent. One research in mice with diabetes also revealed that fasting enhanced persistence proportions and secured against diabetic retinopathy. Diabetic retinopathy is a complication which causes blindness. What this implicates is that intermittent fasting can be very protective for individuals who are in danger of developing type 2 diabetes. Nonetheless, there can be certain differences amongst different genders. One 2005 study on women revealed blood sugar controlling actually degraded during twenty-two-day stretch of intermittent fasting procedures.

## 4. Can Reduce Oxidative Stress and Inflammation in the Body

Increased oxidative stress is one part of getting old, and is a symptom of numerous prolonged diseases. It comprises unbalanced molecules called free radicals. Free radicals react with other essential molecules, such as protein and DNA, and destroy them. Numerous research studies depict that intermittent fasting can enhance the body's resistance to oxidative stress. Furthermore, research shows that intermittent fasting can help fight swelling, another key driver of many common illnesses.

## 5. May Be Beneficial for Heart Health

Illness associated with the heart is, at this time, the world's most prevalent killer. It's widely recognized that several health indicators are linked with either an increase or decrease in danger of heart illness. Intermittent fasting has revealed to better numerous diverse risk aspects, including:

- blood sugar levels
- blood pressure

- blood triglycerides
- total and LDL cholesterol
- swelling

Even more indicators are found in studies on animals. The effects of fasting on heart well-being need to be researched more exhaustively in humans before further endorsements can be made.

## 6. Induces Various Cell Repair Processes

When we fast, the cells in the body start a cellular "waste removal" procedure called autophagy. It encompasses the cells disintegrating and metabolizing broken and dysfunctional proteins that develop inside cells over time. An increase in autophagy may provide a shield against several illnesses, including cancer and neurodegenerative illnesses like Alzheimer's disease.

## 7. May Help in Preventing Tumors

Cancer is caused by uncontrolled cell development. Fasting has exhibited several valuable effects on digestion that may culminate in a reduced risk of cancer. Encouraging evidence from animal research shows that intermittent fasting or foods that copycat fasting may assist in preventing cancer. Research in humans has led to the same findings, although more studies are needed. There's also some evidence presenting that fasting brought down various side effects of chemotherapy in humans.

## 8. Has Benefits for Your Brain

What's good for the body is usually good for the brain also. Intermittent fasting mends various metabolic attributes identified to be essential for brain well-being. Intermittent fasting helps reduce:

- oxidative stress
- inflammation
- blood sugar levels
- insulin resistance

Numerous studies in mice and rats have revealed that intermittent fasting might increase the development of new nerve cells, which should be beneficial for brain health. Fasting also raises levels of a brain hormone called brain-derived neurotrophic factor (BDNF). BDNF insufficiency has been associated with depression and many other brain complications. Animal research has also revealed that intermittent fasting shields against brain damage due to strokes.

## 9. May Prolong Your Lifespan, Helping You Live Longer

The greatest thrilling usage of intermittent fasting is its capacity to prolong the lifespan. Research in rodents shows that intermittent fasting lengthens life in the same way as constant calorie restriction. Fasting has also been shown to increase the lifespans of fruit flies. In some research, the impacts were quite dramatic. In an older research study, rats that were fasted daily lived 83 percent longer than rats who weren't fasted. In a 2017 study, mice that were fasted on a daily basis saw their lifetimes increase by 13 percent. Regular fasting also improved the overall well-being of male mice. It facilitated the delay of the beginning of conditions such as fatty liver illness and hepatocellular carcinoma, which are both common in elderly mice. Even though this is far from being resolved in humans, intermittent fasting has become very common among the antiaging crowd. Taking into account the known gains for metabolism and all kinds of health indicators, it is clear that intermittent fasting could help one live a prolonged and healthier life.

# 2

## YOUR BODY CHANGES IN UNEXPECTED WAYS AFTER 50

You gain wisdom, strength, and experience as you become older. You form significant bonds with those around you and watch them blossom. You start to figure out what matters most to you and let go of some of the restrictions that ruled your younger years. But, in addition to those intangible aspects, your body undergoes changes.

Many of the changes that come with aging are likely familiar to you. For example, your metabolism slows down, making you more prone to high blood pressure and heart disease. You already know not to eat too much salt, and you're probably thinking about restricting foods that can raise your cholesterol. But are there any other, more subtle developments on the horizon?

Everyone ages differently, but there are biological factors that contribute to changes such as wrinkles and graying hair. Other changes, such as those occurring in your brain or at the cellular level, are undetectable. As you approach the second half of your lifespan, you will most likely notice a shift in your feelings. Here are a few of the lesser-known ways your body changes as you get older.

CHANGES

**1. Weight**

Your metabolism slows as you become older. Even while your body is at rest, lean muscles burn calories, but as you get older, your lean muscle mass begins to deteriorate. Your body will begin to accumulate more fat than muscle as a result of this. After fifty, you can offset this by maintaining regular cardiovascular exercise, such as walking or swimming, as well as making lifestyle changes such as eating a more balanced diet and avoiding substances like drugs or nicotine.

After age thirty, it's common to experience an increases in body fat, but men's weight gain typically stops around age fifty-five, while women often continue to gain weight until around age sixty-five. From puberty through menopause, excess weight tends to accumulate around the hips and thighs. However, after that, a woman's excess pounds are more likely to be harmful belly fat, which is linked to a higher risk of heart disease and diabetes.

## 2. Bone Density

For women, bones build density from puberty to adulthood around the age of thirty, especially if you work out frequently and consume a nutritious diet rich in vitamin D and calcium. As hormone levels alter, women begin to experience a loss of bone density gradually around the age of thirty-five, a process that speeds up after menopause. A healthy way of life that includes weight-bearing activities like strength training and walking is beneficial to bone health. The National Osteoporosis Foundation suggests that women have a bone density test at the age of sixty-five, but it's better to obtain one sooner than that. By that age, a woman's lifetime possibility of developing a fragility fracture has already increased to 50 percent.

Drops in estrogen can induce a loss of bone density, putting women over fifty at an increased risk of osteoporosis. According to the National Osteoporosis Foundation, low bone density affects 44 million Americans, with one out of every two women over fifty at risk of breaking a bone due to osteoporosis. Smoking, inactivity, and excessive alcohol use can all harm bone health, but sticking to a well-balanced diet is one of the most effective ways to lower the risk of osteoporosis. Including specific foods that are high in the right nutrients in your diet will help you reduce your risk.

Genetics, gender, age, medical history, and lifestyle choices all have a role in whether or not a person gets osteoporosis. However, the latter is the only issue over which we have control. Smoking, inactivity, and excessive alcohol use can all have an impact on bone health, but sticking to a well-balanced diet is one of the most effective ways to lower the risk of osteoporosis.

Though it's difficult to live a life without hip surgery and bone-related hospital visits, some meals can help with calcium absorption, bone density, and bone strength by supplying sufficient levels of key nutrients including magnesium, vitamin D, protein, and calcium. However, some foods, such as animal proteins, can have a negative impact on bone health by leaking calcium—something you should be aware of. These essential nutrients must therefore originate from the proper sources in order to provide your bones with the strength they require.

## 3. Skin

Women's skin thickness is maintained until they reach the age of fifty. Skin gets thinner, less elastic, and drier as a result, and wrinkles become more visible. Eating a balanced diet, getting lots of restful sleep, drinking plenty of water, and not smoking are all cornerstones of healthy, beautiful skin throughout life, and much more so as you get older. If you want to try natural wrinkle-reduction methods, such as exfoliating and using a retinol night lotion, you can. But what is the most crucial move you can make? Keeping yourself safe from the sun. Your dermatologist may perform a full body scan to search for any abnormalities (such as moles that have changed size or color), but it's also crucial to check yourself once a month.

Watermelon is one food that is particularly hydrating. Water makes up 92 percent of the fruit, while sugar makes up 6 percent. You'd have to eat a little more than a full glass of watermelon to equal one full glass, or 16 ounces by bulk, of water. You'd have drank a whole glass of water if you ate 17.6 ounces of watermelon by volume. That's around three cups of watermelon cubes or two large wedges of the whole fruit.

## 4. Hair Loss or Thinning

If you're going to gray, it'll most likely begin in your thirties, though some women may start sooner (it's entirely genetic). However, as you get older, your hair thins out and grows more slowly. Don't be worried if you've seen additional strands in your brush recently—almost everyone loses hair over time, especially beyond the age of fifty.

Female pattern baldness begins with a widening of the center hair part that spreads to the top and crown of the scalp. It is a hormone-related disorder that can be inherited. Unlike male pattern baldness, it rarely affects a woman's entire head of hair. You can increase the health of your hair regardless of your age or condition by avoiding harsh chemicals and treating it carefully.

Remember that when you go through these and other changes, the passage of time provides a lot of advantages. Many women like the freedom that comes with having children out of the house as they become older, such as not having to worry about birth control. You may also notice a change in your attitude, such as the urge to please people fading away. You may also discover that now is a good moment to reconnect with your actual loves and delights.

To help your hair thrive, you should concentrate on a few crucial nutrients. The first is protein, which is a necessary component of hair cells. The next ingredient is biotin, which boosts your natural keratin storage and promotes healthy hair growth. You should also increase your B vitamin intake, which includes B12, B3, and B5. Vitamins A and C each serve a different role in encouraging healthy blood flow to your scalp, which supports healthy hair development.

Make sure you're consuming plenty in addition to these things. When you're on a calorie-restricted diet, your body isn't going to waste any energy on giving you long, luscious locks. Crash dieters, I apologize.

Eating full, nutritious meals on a daily basis is the best way to encourage hair growth. Topical applications of nourishing mixtures, according to some, may be beneficial. Olive oil, as well as coconut oil and other healthy fats, can help your hair shine. However, regardless of how your hair appears on the outside or how you treat it, eating these nutrients may help you grow more hair faster.

## 5. Changes in Sleep Patterns

Having trouble sleeping like you used to? Don't be alarmed; it's not always an indicator of insomnia. Changes in sleep patterns are a completely natural aspect of the aging process, according to the National Sleep Foundation. You're more likely to sleep less soundly and consistently as you become older. Many elderly people report having trouble falling asleep and waking up several times during the night.

## 6. Heart

Estrogen appears to help keep artery walls flexible and may raise HDL ("good") cholesterol levels while lowering LDL ("bad") cholesterol levels. It also prevents abdominal fat from accumulating, which adds to inflammation, which can raise the risk of a heart attack. Heart disease rates in women increase two to three times after menopause, when estrogen levels drop; more than 75 percent of women aged forty to sixty have one or more risk factors for coronary heart disease. Those who eat a healthy diet, exercise regularly, and don't smoke, on the other hand, are 80 percent less likely than women who don't to acquire heart disease. Follow your doctor's blood pressure and lipid screening recommendations, which will be based on a variety of criteria, such as your age and family history of heart disease.

### 7. Immune System

It may take longer to hunt down viruses and additional harmful agents. Your body is also extra prone to accidentally attacking itself. In addition, your body is no longer able to produce a large number of "fighter" cells to fight toxicities as it once did. As a result of all of this, you're more likely to get ill with tetanus, pneumonia, and the flu, so take precautions and make certain you're current on your vaccinations.

### 8. Muscles

You begin to lose muscle mass at a faster rate after the age of fifty. Physical strength can deteriorate as well. Lifting weights or doing strength training activities like lunges and squats two to three times a week is the best approach to arrest this downward spiral. You'll not only increase your lean muscle mass, but you'll also enhance your balance, which will come in handy as you age.

### 9. Joints

The cartilage and tissues that cushion your joints diminish with age, and you'll notice the impacts in your fifties. Start with your posture to avoid joint pain and arthritis. (Men may notice it sooner.) You put pressure on your joints when you slouch. Also, maintain track of your weight, as excess pounds might put strain on your joints. Drink plenty of water as well. Your body draws fluid from joint tissue when you're thirsty.

## 10. Vision

Because the lenses inside your eyes stiffen as you get older, you may have to squint to view your phone. They can't adjust from a distance focus to an up-close perspective as rapidly as they used to. You could need new glasses (such "readers" that you can get without a prescription) or a new vision prescription. As you get older, your vision will deteriorate, so schedule regular eye checkups.

## 11. Menopause

Women begin to experience menopause at the age of fifty. The ovaries of women begin to generate less estrogen and progesterone and more follicle-stimulating hormone (FSH). The symptoms of hormonal changes differ from person to person, however many women report insomnia, hot flashes, decreased libido, sadness, and mood swings as a result of these changes. Some men, too, are affected by hormonal shifts. According to the Rush University Medical Center, about 20 percent of men over the age of sixty go through andropause, which is marked by a reduction in testosterone production. Lowered energy levels, depression, decreased muscle strength, and diminished sex drive are just a few of the symptoms.

## 12. Bladder Control

Strong muscles and ligaments that support your pelvic floor are essential for your sexual, reproductive, and urinary health. Changes in the body caused by childbearing, menopause, and hysterectomies all can affect women's health, especially involving pelvic organ prolapse (when the pelvic organs fall out of position), and urine incontinence, which is the inability to regulate urination. Preventing these problems can be as simple as maintaining pelvic-floor and core strength. Kegels, the most basic pelvic floor exercise, are straightforward: Pretend you're holding in gas for ten seconds with an empty bladder, then relax for ten seconds. Three to five times a day, do five to ten reps. Menopause also causes vaginal tissue to shrink and dry, making sex less pleasurable.

## 13. Color Perception

Even if you were never color-blind, once you reach the age of fifty, you may lose your capacity to discern between different colours. Your eyes' clear lenses may begin to dim, interfering with your ability to perceive colors, according to the American Optometric Association.

## 14. Sweat with an Unusual Odor

There's a biological reason for the reported "old people" odor. Hormonal changes might cause a change in the makeup of your sweat as you get older. Furthermore, some studies reveal that as people get older, their bodies produce more 2-Nonenal, a chemical that adds to body odor.

## 15. Sense of Flavor

Your perception of taste may deteriorate with age, but not because of your taste buds, according to the National Institute of Aging. This shift is due in large part to your sense of smell, which influences your capacity to taste food. Medications can sometimes cause taste problems as a side effect. This is even more incentive to savor all of your guilty pleasure meals while they're still fresh in your mind.

## 16. Ability to Recall Memories

As we get older, some memory changes are to be expected. It's possible that you've noticed that remembering new knowledge is becoming more difficult. Long-term memory, the ability to do familiar activities, and retrieving general knowledge are all memory functions that don't alter greatly with age. Certain meals can help you combat memory loss in the same way they can aid your physical health.

Everyone experiences memory lapses from time to time. Memory loss, on the other hand, can be a serious medical issue for some people. When memory loss begins to interfere with your daily life, it may be an unnoticed signal of a severe condition such as Alzheimer's or dementia. Fortunately, there are certain things you can do to reduce your chance of not only those diseases, but also memory loss as you become older.

Exercise, according to doctors, is one of the most effective ways to prevent Alzheimer's disease. According to the Alzheimer's

Association, other lifestyle adjustments that may help include reading every day, keeping up with your social life, stopping smoking, and getting adequate sleep. However, your food plays a part as well. Eating more nutrient-dense foods may help you fight memory loss.

## 17. Teeth

According to Harvard Health, your risks of significant tooth damage or root canal therapy triple beyond the age of sixty-five. Years of biting, grinding, and gnawing eat away the outer layer of enamel, making your teeth more vulnerable to dental concerns including cracks, breaks, and infections. Commit to frequent dental visits to avoid tooth decay. There is no predetermined number of visits each year; you should see your dentist as often as they deem fit.

## 18. Digestive System

As you become older, a few things affect your digestion. Because your stomach produces less acid, certain drugs and vitamin absorption may be more challenging. The muscles in your esophagus and bowels may also slow down, producing digestion issues such as acid reflux and constipation. Fortunately, there are a few teas that can help you feel better.

Tea is a great way to warm up on a cold day, and if you drink it often, it may even save you from becoming sick. Many teas include important micronutrients that can help you avoid cancer, heart disease, and diabetes, as well as boost your immune system and relieve stomach aches. These teas may help quiet your upset stomach if you're experiencing digestive troubles, but they're not a cure-all.

## 19. Breasts

After adolescence, breasts change slowly, and each menstrual period can bring about temporary changes. The milk duct system swells to nurse a baby, therefore the breasts swell during pregnancy. As estrogen levels drop after menopause, the breasts alter again, becoming less plump and less elastic, which can lead to "sagging." Breast cancer risk rises with age, despite the fact that a thirty-year-old woman's ten-year risk of getting breast cancer is 1 in 227, a sixty-year-old woman's ten-year risk is 1 in 28. Although genetics play a part in breast cancer, you can minimize your risk by maintaining a healthy body weight, exercising regularly, limiting your alcohol intake, and using hormone replacement treatment for less than five years if you need it. Every year, all women aged fifty and over should receive a mammogram.

## 20. Stress

There's no denying that navigating the changes of midlife can be stressful. We'd all prefer to be less stressed in our daily lives. Stress, on the other hand, can be beneficial because it keeps us alert. When we are constantly confronted with obstacles with no end in sight, stress develops. Tension builds up in the body, resulting in a variety of physical issues such as headaches, indigestion, high blood pressure, chest discomfort, and insomnia.

The consequences of persistent stress are amplified in women over fifty. Because your body isn't as tough as it once was, it requires greater care—a healthier lifestyle—in order to heal. It's time to admit it: it's time to relax.

What are the secrets to reducing stress and increasing happiness? According to Charles Raison, MD, they aren't more money or material items. Positive activity, good health, excellent relationships, and a sense of optimism are the four pillars.

## How to Achieve Emotional Balance and Reduce Stress

1. **Exercise often.** Exercise lowers stress levels, promotes happiness, and improves general health. It also aids in better sleep.
2. **Build a support structure.** Becoming a member of a religious community can help some people cope with stress. For others, joining a swim club or a sewing circle may be the answer. Solid friendships, though, can help you experience warmth, stability, and connection no matter where you discover them.
3. **Keep a positive approach.** Look for the bright side and excellent news. Make a list of things for which you are grateful.

4. **Avoid negativity.** Accept that there are some things over which you have no control.
5. **Be firm instead of hostile.** Assert your feelings, thoughts, or beliefs rather than getting angry, defensive, or passive.
6. **Discover new desires.** Having a feeling of adventure can aid with stress reduction. Pay attention to your dreams. Find something to feel enthusiastic about. Make a hobby out of it. Be inventive!

# 3

## CHOOSING THE RIGHT TYPE OF FASTING

In recent years, fasting on a regular basis has proven to be beneficial and has become a fashionable health craze. It is said by devotees that it can assist people in losing weight, improving metabolic well-being, and possibly even extending their lives. Every method has the potential to be beneficial. Choosing which one, though, is a challenge. It is a personal choice. There are several methods to approach this way of eating. However, before starting and determining how often to fast on an intermittent basis, you should consult with a healthcare professional. Intermittent fasting can be done in five different ways.

## 1. WHAT IS 16/8 INTERMITTENT FASTING?

The 16/8 method of intermittent fasting is restricting food and consumption of calorie-containing drinks to an eight-hour window per day, and fasting for the remaining sixteen hours. This cycle can be performed as often as you'd like, anywhere from once or twice a week to every day, depending on your preferences. In recent years, 16/8 intermittent fasting has exploded in popularity, especially among individuals wanting to reduce weight and burn fat. Other diets have rigorous rules and regulations, but 16/8 intermittent fasting is simple to follow and can yield substantial results with little effort. It's widely regarded as being less restrictive and more adaptable than many other diet programs, and it may easily fit into almost any lifestyle. This method of intermittent fasting is thought to increase blood sugar regulation, brain function, and longevity in addition to promoting weight loss.

### How To Get Started

The 16/8 method of intermittent fasting is simple, safe, and long-term. To begin, choose an eight-hour window and restrict your food consumption to that time frame. Many people prefer to eat between midday and 8 p.m., since it allows them to consume a healthy lunch and supper, as well as a few snacks during the day, while just fasting overnight and skipping breakfast. Others choose to eat between the hours of 9 a.m. and 5 p.m., providing enough time for a good breakfast, a regular lunch around midday, and, before starting their fast, a light early meal or snack at 4 p.m. You can, however, experiment to find the time range that works best for you. To maximize the health benefits of your diet, it's also critical to stick to healthy whole foods and beverages during mealtimes. Consuming nutrient-dense meals can help fill out your diet and allow you to gain the benefits of this routine. Try to include a range of healthful whole foods in each meal, such as:

- **Fruits**: such as pears, peaches, oranges, berries, bananas, and apples.
- **Veggies**: such as tomatoes, leafy greens, cucumbers, cauliflower, and broccoli.
- **Whole grains**: such as buckwheat, barley, oats, rice, and quinoa.
- **Healthy fats**: such as avocados, coconut oil, and olive oil.
- **Sources of protein**: like seeds, nuts, eggs, legumes, fish, poultry, and meat.

Even during fasting, calorie-free beverages such as water, unsweetened tea, and coffee can help manage your appetite while keeping you hydrated. Binging or overdoing it on junk food, on the other hand, might counteract the benefits of 16/8 intermittent fasting and cause more harm than good to your health.

## Benefits of 16/8 Intermittent Fasting

The 16/8 method of intermittent fasting is a popular diet because it is simple to follow, adaptable, and sustainable in the long-term. It's also convenient because it can help you save time and money by reducing the amount of time and money you spend cooking and preparing food each week. In terms of health, this method of intermittent fasting has been linked to a slew of advantages, including:

- **Increased weight reduction:** Not only does limiting your consumption to a few hours each day help you burn calories throughout the day, but studies show that this method of fasting can also accelerate your metabolism and help you lose weight.
- **Improved Blood Sugar Management:** This method of fasting has been shown to reduce fasting insulin levels by up to 31 percent and blood sugar levels by 3–6 percent, potentially lowering your diabetes risk.
- **Prolonged Life Expectancy:** Though there is little proof in humans, certain animal studies have suggested that 16/8 fasting can help people live longer.

## Drawbacks of 16/8 Intermittent Fasting

This method of intermittent fasting has a number of health benefits, but it also has certain negatives and may not be suitable for everyone. Some people may eat more than usual during eating periods to make up for hours spent fasting if they limit their intake to only eight hours per day. Weight gain, digestive issues, and the development of poor eating habits are all possible outcomes. When you first start 16/8 intermittent fasting, you may experience short-term unpleasant side effects including hunger, weakness, and exhaustion, but these usually fade once you get into a routine. Furthermore, some evidence suggests that intermittent fasting has different effects on men and women, with animal studies indicating that it may interfere with female fertility and reproduction. More human research is needed, however, to determine the impact of intermittent fasting on reproductive health. In any event, start slowly and stop or visit your doctor if you have any concerns or negative side effects.

## 2. WHAT IS 5:2 INTERMITTENT FASTING?

The 5:2 method of intermittent fasting is a type of diet that involves fasting on a regular basis. The Fast Diet, often known as the 5:2 diet, is the most popular intermittent fasting diet at the moment. Michael Mosley, a British journalist, popularized it. The 5:2 diet takes its name from the fact that you can eat normally five days a week, while restricting yourself to 500–600 calories on the other two days. This diet is more of a lifestyle than a diet because there are no restrictions on what foods you can consume, only when you should eat them. Many people find this style of eating to be simpler to keep to than a standard calorie-restricted diet.

## How To Do the 5:2 Diet

It's actually quite simple to ascribe to the 5:2 diet. You eat regularly for five days a week and don't have to worry about calorie restriction. Then you cut your calorie consumption to a quarter of your daily requirements on the other two days. This equates to roughly 500 calories per day for women and 600 calories per day for men. You are at liberty to fast on any two days of the week so long as you have, at the very least, one non-fasting day in the middle. Fasting on Mondays and Thursdays with two or three modest meals, then eating regularly for the rest of the week, is a common way of arranging the week. It's crucial to note that eating "normally" does not imply that you can eat whatever you want. If you eat junk food in excess, you are unlikely to lose weight and may even gain weight. You should eat as much as you would if you weren't fasting at all.

## Benefits of 5:2 Intermittent Fasting

There are very few studies particularly on the 5:2 diet. There is, however, numerous research on intermittent fasting in general that demonstrates significant health benefits. Intermittent fasting, at least for some people, has the advantage of being simpler to stick to than continuous calorie restriction. In addition, many studies have demonstrated that various types of intermittent fasting can lower insulin levels dramatically. According to one study, the 5:2 diet helped people lose weight in the same way that calorie restriction did. Furthermore, the diet was particularly successful in lowering insulin levels and boosting insulin sensitivity. The health effects of modified alternate-day fasting, which is comparable to the 5:2 diet, have been cited in several studies. Insulin resistance, asthma, seasonal allergies, cardiac arrhythmias, menopausal hot flashes, and other conditions may be helped by the 5:2 diet.

When compared to a control group that ate regularly, the group undertaking 5:2 fasting showed significant improvements in both normal-weight and overweight persons. The fasting group got the following results after twelve weeks:

- Body weight was reduced by more than 11 pounds (5 kg).
- Lost 7.7 pounds (3.5 kg) of fat mass while maintaining muscle mass.
- Triglyceride levels in the blood were reduced by 20 percent.
- LDL particle size had increased, which was a favorable sign.
- CRP levels, an essential inflammatory marker, were lower.
- Leptin levels were reduced by as much as 40 percent.

## Drawbacks of 5:2 Intermittent Fasting

- **Difficult acclimation phase:** While the 5:2 diet may be sustainable once you've gotten acclimated to it, it does necessitate some major commitment at first. During the first few fasts, you'll probably experience intense hunger as well as other negative symptoms such as exhaustion and irritation. However, once you've gotten beyond the initial side effects, your body should adjust and you should feel back to normal.
- **Danger of overeating:** Calorie restriction always carries the risk of overeating. Not only can this lead to the unpleasant side effects of overeating, but it may also prevent you from achieving your health or weight-loss goals.

## 3. WHAT IS EAT STOP EAT INTERMITTENT FASTING?

The Eat Stop Eat method of intermittent fasting has become very popular. It's similar to the 5:2 method, where fasting is restricted to only one or two days a week, but the fasting days are ones in which you do not consume any calories at all. Below, we'll dive into how to do it, as well as its benefits and potential drawbacks.

## How To Do the Eat Stop Eat Diet

The Eat Stop Eat diet is simple to follow. You just go without eating or fasting for a complete twenty-four-hour period on one or two nonconsecutive days every week. The remaining five to six days of the week are yours to eat as much as you like, but it's recommended that you make prudent food choices and don't consume more than your body requires. When you utilize the Eat Stop Eat approach, you will still consume something on each calendar day of the week, which may seem irrational. If you're fasting from 9 a.m. Tuesday to 9 a.m. Wednesday, for example, you'll consume something before 9 a.m. Tuesday. On Wednesday, after 9 a.m., you'll have your next meal. This ensures that you fast for the whole twenty-four hours, but no longer. Keep in mind that regular water is recommended even on Eat Stop Eat fasting days. Drinking a lot of water is the best option, however, calorie-free beverages such as sugar-free coffee or tea are also allowed.

## Benefits of Eat Stop Eat Intermittent Fasting

### 1. May encourage weight loss

Weight loss is one of the primary motivations for people to try intermittent fasting diets like Eat Stop Eat. Though there are presently no trials assessing Eat Stop Eat for weight loss, accumulating data suggests that the intermittent, protracted fasting used by Eat Stop Eat may help some people lose weight.

## 2. Calorie Deficit

A calorie deficit is the first—and arguably most evident—method that Eat Stop Eat can help you to lose weight. It's common knowledge that losing weight necessitates consuming fewer calories than you burn. Eat Stop Eat, when used correctly, sets you up for a calorie deficit of one to two days each week. This decrease in overall calorie intake may result in weight loss over time as you burn more calories than you consume. However, recent evidence suggests that calorie restriction for a whole day is no more helpful for weight loss than the continuous daily calorie restriction used by most traditional diets.

## 3. Metabolic Shifts

Another reason Eat Stop Eat may help you lose weight is because of metabolic changes that occur when your body is starved. Carbohydrates are the body's preferred fuel source. Carbs are broken down into a useful kind of energy called glucose when you eat them. Most people will burn up the glucose they have stored in their bodies after twelve to thirty-six hours of fasting, and will then switch to using fat as an energy source. Ketosis is the metabolic state in which this occurs. According to preliminary studies, prolonged fasting may boost fat use in a way that typical dieting regimens cannot. Still, there isn't much research on this possible advantage, and there appears to be a lot of variation in how rapidly people enter ketosis. As a result, it's doubtful that everyone will achieve ketosis within the Eat Stop Eat diet's twenty-four-hour fasting window. More research is needed to better understand how metabolic changes caused by the Eat Stop Eat diet can affect fat loss and overall weight loss.

## Drawbacks of Eat Stop Eat Intermittent Fasting

For most healthy adults, the fasting procedures used in Eat Stop Eat are probably safe. However, if you're considering about trying it out, you should think about the following drawbacks:

### 1. Insufficient Nutrient Intake

> On the Eat Stop Eat diet, some people may struggle to meet all of their nutritional demands. It's not uncommon for people to think about food solely in terms of calories when they're dieting. Food, on the other hand, is much more than just calories. It's also high in vitamins, minerals, and other helpful substances that help support your body's most crucial activities. Anyone who is paying attention to Eat Stop Eat must pay extra thoughtfulness to the items they consume on their non-fasting days in order to maintain adequate vitamin, fiber, protein, and mineral intake during the course of their diet. If you have extremely high nutritional needs or are currently unable to eat enough food to meet them, eliminating one to two days' worth of food may result in nutrient deficiency or unhealthy weight loss.

## 2. Low Blood Sugar

Intermittent fasting regimens such as Eat Stop Eat are used by some people to enhance blood sugar control and insulin sensitivity. Most healthy people have no trouble sustaining blood sugar levels during the Eat Stop Eat twenty-four-hour fasting intervals, but this isn't true for everyone. Extended durations without food can cause significant blood sugar decreases, which can be life-threatening in some people, such as diabetics. Consult a healthcare professional before undertaking Eat Stop Eat or any other diet that includes fasting if you take blood sugar medications or have any medical issues that cause poor blood sugar regulation.

## 3. Hormonal changes

The Eat Stop Eat diet's fasting practices may cause changes in metabolic and reproductive hormone production. However, due to a dearth of human research, the particular health implications resulting from such hormonal alterations are difficult to predict. Some research suggests that hormonal alterations may have beneficial health benefits, such as better fertility, while others show a danger of negative consequences, such as insufficient reproductive hormone production and pregnancy difficulties. Eat Stop Eat is not generally recommended for anyone who is pregnant, lactating, or trying to conceive due to the mixed results and low total evidence. Consult a healthcare professional before beginning the Eat Stop Eat regimen if you have a history of hormone deregulation, irregular periods, or amenorrhea.

## 4. Psychological Impact of Restrictive Eating

While many people claim that fasting as a weight-loss strategy gives them greater dietary freedom, the limited nature of such eating patterns may have a negative psychological impact. According to some studies, fasting for a short period of time might cause irritation, mood swings, and a decrease in libido. However, proponents of intermittent fasting frequently claim that mood troubles go away as you become used to your fasting regimen—but this has yet to be confirmed. Restrictive dieting can lead to disordered eating habits including binge eating or obsessive thoughts about food and weight. Eat Stop Eat is therefore not recommended for anyone with a history of disordered eating or a proclivity to develop these behaviours.

## 4. WHAT IS ALTERNATE-DAY FASTING?

Intermittent fasting can be done in a variety of ways, including alternate-day fasting. You fast every other day on this regimen, but eat whatever you want on the non-fasting days. The most popular variation of this diet is "modified" fasting, which allows you to eat roughly 500 calories on fasting days. Fasting on alternate days can help you lose weight and reduce your risk of heart disease and type 2 diabetes. Here's a step-by-step introduction to alternate-day fasting for beginners.

### How To Do Alternate-Day Fasting

Fasting on alternate days is a type of intermittent fasting. The main concept is that you fast one day and eat whatever you want on the following day. This way, you just have to limit your food intake half of the time. On fasting days, you can consume beverages that are free from calories as you desire, such as water and unsweetened tea and coffee.

On days when you are fasting, you're also allowed to eat about 500 calories, or 20–25 percent of your energy requirements, if you're following a modified ADF approach. Dr. Krista Varady, who has conducted the majority of the studies on alternate day fasting, has created the most popular variant of this diet, dubbed "The Every Other Day Diet." Whether the fasting-day calories are ingested at lunch or supper, or as small meals throughout the day, the rewards of well-being and weight reduction appear to be similar. Alternate-day fasting may be simpler to stick to for some people than other diets.

However, adherence to alternate-day fasting (in which calorie intake is cut to 25 percent of energy demands on fasting days) was not found to be superior to daily calorie restriction in a yearlong trial. The modified form, with 500 calories on fasting days, was employed in the majority of investigations on alternate-day fasting. This is believed to be far more maintainable than complete fasts on fasting days, but it is equally beneficial. The phrases "alternate-day fasting" are used in this text to refer to a modified strategy with roughly 500 calories on fasting days.

## Benefits of Alternate-Day Fasting

Aside from weight loss, alternate-day fasting has a number of health benefits.

## 1. Type 2 Diabetes

In the United States, type 2 diabetes accounts for 90–95 percent of diabetes cases. Furthermore, more than a third of Americans suffer from prediabetes, a condition in which blood sugar levels are above normal but not high enough to be categorized as diabetes. Many of the symptoms of type 2 diabetes can be improved or reversed by losing weight and controlling calories. Alternate-day fasting appears to provide mild decreases in risk variables for type 2 diabetes in adults who are overweight or obese, similar to continuous calorie restriction. Alternate-day fasting may also help lower fasting insulin levels, with some research suggesting that it is more beneficial than calorie restriction on a daily basis. However, not all research agrees that alternate-day fasting is better than calorie restriction on a daily basis. Obesity and chronic diseases, including heart disease and cancer, have been related to having high insulin levels or hyperinsulinemia. Reduced insulin levels and insulin resistance, especially when accompanied with weight loss, should result in a much lower risk of type 2 diabetes.

## 2. Heart Health

Heart disease is the major cause of death worldwide, accounting for one out of every four deaths. Many studies have indicated that alternate-day fasting can assist people who are overweight or obese lose weight and lower their heart disease risk factors. These studies vary from eight to fifty-two weeks, and their participants are overweight or obese. The most common health advantages are:

- A smaller waist circumference (between 2 and 2.8 inches or 5 and 7 cm).
- Reduced LDL (bad) cholesterol by 20–25 percent.
- A growth in the amount of large LDL particles, but the number of harmful small, dense LDL particles decreased.
- Lower triglyceride levels in the blood (up to 30 percent).

## Drawbacks of Alternating-Day Fasting

- Cravings and hunger is one of the most common negative effects of alternate-day fasting, which comes as no surprise.
- Lightheadedness and headaches.
- Digestive problems.
- Irritability as well as other mood swings.
- Tiredness and a lack of energy.
- Nasty breath.
- Sleep disruptions.
- Dehydration.

## 5. WHAT IS 12:12 INTERMITTENT FASTING?

If you're new to fasting, this is a great place to start. Consider it a comparable overnight fast to what you'd do before a blood test. If your doctor has arranged a blood test for the next morning, you may be told to stop eating after dinner and not eat again until the morning of the test. Keeping a twelve-hour fast doesn't get any easier than that.

## How To Do 12:12 Intermittent Fasting

If you fast for twelve hours, your day will be cut in half. You'll eat all of your calories in a twelve-hour period and then fast for another twelve-hour period. This technique aims to help you become acclimated to fasting. You may learn about intermittent fasting and think it sounds great, but when it comes time to put it into practice, you may have concerns:

- Will I go hungry? Will I become unwell as a result of this?
- Will going without food for the remainder of the day cause me to binge?

It's natural to be nervous when you first begin intermittent fasting. Fasting for twelve hours can help you overcome your fears and acquire confidence. It becomes considerably easier when you fast during the hours you sleep. Start by eating your dinner as you normally would. You will not require an additional meal to get you through the night. Take note of the last time you ate—this is the start of your fast. Drink some water or tea before going to bed, but don't eat or drink anything caloric. If you're having trouble avoiding late-night munching, try brushing your teeth. Your tongue will feel clean and fresh, which may help you resist hunger and make you reconsider placing more food on it. You may have your regular breakfast after twelve hours to break your fast. You've completed the task! The only thing left is to keep track of your emotions.

## Benefits of 12:12 Intermittent Fasting

You may eat three or more meals during the day as usual, as long as your calorie consumption is limited to a twelve-hour period. It's very easy to acclimate to this method of intermittent fasting.

## Drawbacks of 12:12 Intermittent Fasting

While this brief period without food may help to maintain weight and control blood sugar levels, it will not provide the total weight-loss and health benefits of other intermittent fasting methods.

# 4

# THE DOS AND DON'TS OF INTERMITTENT FASTING

Intermittent fasting isn't for everyone, and the benefits aren't universal. Given your health, commitment level, and other lifestyle characteristics, it's critical to carefully examine what's best for you. These dos and don'ts will assist you.

## THE DOS

**Check with your doctor.**

Your doctor may recommend a different sort of diet if you have underlying health issues or are on certain medications. When it comes to the safety of intermittent fasting, it has the potential to harm your health. People with low blood sugar, for example, need glucose all day, and fasting for extended periods of time might be fatal.

**Have a plan.**

You must have a strategy in order for anything you want to accomplish to succeed. Intermittent fasting falls under the same rule. To establish a strategy, you'll need clearly stated objectives and reasons for fasting in the first place. You must also take into account elements specific to your body, such as existing health concerns, in order to ensure that your strategy is precise enough to ensure that the method is effective for you. Before you embark on any diet plan or begin intermittent fasting, have an appointment with your doctor to seek their advice.

**Establish when your eating and fasting intervals will be.**

Fasting can be done in a variety of ways. The following are some of the most popular ways to begin intermittent fasting:

- The 16/8 method: fast for sixteen hours and then eat for eight.
- The 5:2 method: eat normally for five days out of the week, and fast for two.
- The Eat Stop Eat method: fast for twenty-four hours at a time, but eat for every calendar day.
- Alternate-Day fasting: fast every other day.
- The 12:12 method: fasting daily, for twelve hours at a time, and eating during the other twelve hours.

## Get your mind, body, and home in order.

Make sure you're well-rested and emotionally prepared before fasting. It's also a fantastic opportunity to get your house in order, in addition to cleaning your thoughts. Remove any tempting meals or beverages from your kitchen that aren't in line with your fasting aims.

## Transition slowly.

Make sure you're not embarking on an intermittent fasting regimen without first planning ahead of time and thoroughly researching various intermittent fasting protocols. You could want to ease into it by completing the 16/8 regimen a couple of times a week rather than every day, or by starting with a twelve-hour fast and gradually increasing to sixteen hours.

## Drink plenty of fluids.

Because you're going to deprive yourself of meals, you'll need to stay hydrated. During intermittent fasting, it is critical to drink plenty of water. When you ask a professional nutritionist, "What can I drink while fasting?" the first answer you will get is "water." Those on a moderate fast should only consume non-caloric beverages, while those on an open fast should avoid beverages with more than 20 calories.

While fasting, water aids in the feeling of fullness in your stomach, hence reducing hunger. On a regular day, you'd drink a couple glasses of water, and the food you consume also contains water, which helps you stay hydrated. When fasting, drinking more water helps to compensate for the water deficit caused by the lack of meals consumed, allowing you to keep hydrated while on an intermittent fasting journey.

**Make the right food choices.**

Making healthy food choices is the other trick. Fasting may not be able to reverse the effects of a poor diet. You're unlikely to see the results you want if you fast for sixteen hours and then consume pizza and cheeseburgers for the next eight.

**Eat fibrous and fatty foods.**

Fiber-rich foods are more filling, and when combined with foods high in healthy fats, they will keep you satiated for longer.

**Take your vitamins.**

Depending on the type of fast you're undertaking, you may need to supplement with most or all of the vitamins your body requires. Vitamins in liquid form are easier to digest during a fast. Take a multivitamin and calcium supplement separately. It's critical to supplement the vitamins and minerals you'll be losing while fasting because you'll be missing so many.

LIPO-DREX, for example, can help you lose weight faster. This fat-burning supplement might help you get the most out of intermittent fasting. Unlike other fat loss supplements, iSatori's LIPO-DREX encourages fat reduction without the muscle loss that is sometimes an unwelcome side effect of weight loss.

LIPO-DREX employs a novel mechanism known as nutrient partitioning. Nutrients are delivered directly to the muscles rather than being deposited in fat cells as a result of nutrition partitioning. This translates to a speedier leaning-out process, with stronger muscles and more energy.

**Pay attention to your body.**

Because everyone's body reacts to fasting differently, there's no way to know how you'll react until you've started fasting. When you begin fasting, pay attention to any changes in your body, energy levels, or any other undesirable symptoms that may develop. Stop the fast as soon as you feel weak, disoriented, or unable to carry out your normal daily activities. When you initially begin fasting, you may feel weary or sluggish because your body is working with less energy than it is used to. If you continue to feel this way, you should consider breaking your fast or obtaining medical counsel from your doctor.

**Incorporate your fast into your day-to-day routine**

Before you go on a fast, think about it. Fasting should be avoided at times of high stress. Start the process when you're not under a lot of pressure. Starting an intermittent fasting program can come with its own set of challenges. For example, you will first be preoccupied with when you will be able to eat. Keeping your goals in mind can help you manage this. This will also assist you in staying on pace for success.

## Make an effort to find enjoyable distractions.

So it's possible that you won't be able to eat chocolate while fasting. That isn't to say you can't enjoy other activities. Get a massage or a mani-pedi, or take a stroll through the mall and do some window shopping. It's also a good idea to stay away from hunger triggers. Don't go grocery shopping or out to supper with pals just to watch them eat. Avoid all of the mouth-wateringly appealing food photographs on social media.

## Get help from your friends.

Making a phone call to a friend can help you get through your fast without going insane. Even better, enlist the help of a buddy or your partner. Isn't anyone interested? Look for internet support groups to find other people who are going through the same thing as you. Developing accountability is a powerful strategy for achieving success. While you may not be consuming the same items because everyone's nutrient requirements differ, sending—or getting—a motivational text in the thirteenth hour of a fast can be extremely helpful.

## Accept the fact that you will be hungry during your fast.

Intermittent fasting causes hunger. The good news is that you will learn to control and lessen fasting window hunger with time. From drinking plenty of water or a cup of black coffee, to learning how to resist food temptations and scheduling busy meetings or exercises during the fasting window, there are many things you may do to stay on track. There are several options for getting through some difficult fasting hours. All you have to do now is figure out what works best for you.

**Take pleasure in your intermittent fasting experience.**

While weight loss is a tremendous benefit of intermittent fasting, taking control of your urges is also an empowering sensation. Many people also claim to be more focused, invigorated, sleep better, and, of course, feel and look better. Even after only a few weeks of intermittent fasting, these improvements are noticeable.

Intermittent fasting can become a crucial part of one's daily routine, and it shouldn't be a source of anxiety. As a result, it's critical to figure out what type of intermittent fasting schedule works best for you and how to avoid adverse effects, lessen hunger, and yet eat a nutritious, balanced diet to fuel your body.

**Concentrate on your objectives.**

It will take some time to adjust to intermittent fasting, so keep yourself busy and focused on why you're fasting in the first place. Consider why you want to reduce weight when hunger sensations come. Is it to feel better about yourself? To have a slimmer figure? To squeeze into those new jeans? In order to get your attention off the desires, concentrate on your goals.

## THE DON'TS

### Start with an extreme plan.

Don't you want to jump in with all your excitement and, well, kick the crap out of it now that you've found a fasting strategy that sounds just right for your needs? You're probably already envisioning your new look once you've lost the weight. Is it possible to begin fasting right now? No, no, allowing your zeal to lead you to an intense strategy that will drastically alter your physique is not a good idea. You can't go from three meals a day plus snacks to a twenty-four-hour fast. You will be miserable as a result of this. Begin by skipping individual meals. Alternatively, avoiding snacking. Once your body has become accustomed to short fasts, you can go as far as your body will allow, within reason. Exercise slowly during the fasting phase, at least in the first several weeks, as this can lead to adrenal fatigue.

### Eat too much the day before fasting.

When you know you won't be eating much, if anything, the next day, you might be tempted to overeat the night before. It's important to refuel for the next day, but fatty foods should be avoided. Your body requires slow-burning nutrients to keep you energized throughout the day, so choose nutrient-dense foods like carbs, proteins, and unsaturated fats.

**Break the fast too rapidly.**

It's also crucial to keep track of how much food you eat following a fast. Break the fast with a small, nutrient-dense snack. Do not eat a large dinner soon after fasting because you are prone to eat more than you require.

**Quit too soon.**

Have you only been fasting for a week and already think it's too difficult? Do you have hunger pangs, cravings, mood swings, low energy, and other issues? Such a reaction is to be expected, after all. As the body adjusts to the lower calorie intake, the first few weeks might be difficult. You'll be famished, irritated, and tired. You must, however, maintain your consistency. The body is adapting to the changes, even if you can't feel it. If you quit during this time and go back to your old eating habits, you'll undo the changes your body has already made. Any change, including this one, necessitates discipline. Keep your chin up; things will improve with time.

**Fast if you have a medical issue.**

Fasting isn't suitable for everyone. Your body requires all the energy it can get if you have a chronic condition, are pregnant, or are taking medication. Fasting deprives the body of this energy, making it unwise to embark on a fasting regimen. While intermittent fasting is mainly a weight-loss and weight-maintenance approach, there are alternative weight-loss methods that may be better suited to your needs. Consult your doctor for recommendations on which weight-loss procedures are best for you.

**Ignore what your body is telling you.**

Even if your doctor has given you permission to attempt intermittent fasting, your body may tell you that it isn't right for you. If you're having extreme headaches, stomach upset, low energy, and dizziness as a result of your diet program, it's time to call it quits or, at the very least, reconsider your approach. When it comes to your workouts while undergoing intermittent fasting, you need to listen to your body. If your body hasn't been adequately fuelled, certain workouts, such as high-intensity interval training or Crossfit training, may be too difficult to complete. It's possible you'll need to ease up on yourself on fasting days, or modify your workout timing to ensure you have enough stamina to get through it.

**Treat your non-fasting period as a buffet.**

You may not see benefits if you overeat during your eating window and consume more calories than you need. When you're not fasting, one of the keys to intermittent fasting success is eating within a sensible calorie range. Learn how to keep your body burning fat by increasing your metabolic rate. Binge eating and empty calorie items and snacks should be avoided.

## Limit your calorie intake during the eating phase.

The eating period's goal is to provide your body with the energy it requires to function. It's tempting to limit calories at this time, but doing so can sabotage your progress and drive your body to seek more food, causing you to break your fast before you're ready.

## Binge-eat during the eating phase.

Binging is the polar opposite of calorie restriction. This can also be harmful because it will increase calorie consumption and so reduce the benefits of fasting.

## Overwork your body during the fasting phase.

When you fast, your body is deprived of the energy it normally receives from your daily meals. While it's fine to work out as usual, it's critical not to overwork your body to the point of exhaustion.

## Participate in tasks that require a lot of energy during your fast.

You must balance nutrition with exercise if you are to lose weight or at least maintain the weight loss you have already accomplished. However, exercising or indulging in intensive activities while fasting is not recommended. Light to moderate exercise has been shown in studies to be more beneficial than severe exercise. Overdoing it can have a bad impact on your body and your mental state, making it more difficult to stick to your fasting schedule. At the same time, don't let the fact that you're fasting serve as an excuse to do nothing.

**Try to be a hero.**

Fasting has major consequences, so pay attention to your body and stop if you feel you're pushing yourself too hard or too far. Symptoms such as dizziness, weakness, and heart palpitations should be taken seriously. Stop immediately if you're feeling bad. You should pay attention to your body and keep in mind that fasting isn't the ideal option for everyone. If you're not feeling well, use common sense and break the fast.

**Go for the burn.**

Are you considering running a marathon or a 5K? It's not a good idea to do it while you're fasting. While mild exercise is good, high-intensity activities should be avoided. Examine your schedule to ensure that you don't have any high-intensity activities scheduled on fasting days, as this will jeopardize your ability to stick to your fast.

**Victory binge.**

After the fast, refrain from overindulging. Instead, gradually return to a healthy habit. Eat three little or five to six micromeals per day to keep your weight down. Avoid meals that are difficult to digest, such as cruciferous vegetables, and gradually reintroduce high-fiber foods. If you drink alcohol, be particularly cautious. It's fine to consume a small amount of alcohol, and you can drink alcohol during an eating window, such as a glass of wine, but not on an empty stomach. When breaking a fast, you also don't want to drink first thing.

**Pay attention to the time.**

While it's important to make sure you're fasting for the right period of time, don't let it consume your life. If you want to change your perspective about food and how often you should eat, try setting a timer on your phone to remind you when it's time to eat again.

**Make yourself uncomfortable.**

At first, intermittent fasting can be difficult on your body, especially if you're used to eating six to eight little meals throughout the day. Another reason why you might perform better switching to eating fewer meals during the day and then switching up the hours to follow an intermittent fasting diet is because of this. If you feel faint after going too long without eating, it's time to rethink your intermittent fasting routine.

**Work out too hard.**

While high-intensity activities should be avoided when you're fasting, low- to moderate-intensity exercise could be useful. In one study, moderate exercise and eating 20 to 25 percent of calories for two days a week resulted in more weight loss than fasting or exercising alone. However, you must consume at least

25 percent of your daily calories in order to avoid losing muscle mass.

## Be inconsistent with your intermittent fasting routine.

In intermittent fasting, consistency is crucial. It will be easier to implement intermittent fasting into your life if you stick to the same fasting window each day. It will become a habit that will become a part of your daily routine, increasing your chances of sticking to it and succeeding.

Of course, our daily lives are unexpected at times, and plans can alter. Don't give up—just get back on track the next day. It's extremely vital in these situations to have a routine that you've already established and that works for you.

## Consume zero-calorie drinks and artificial sweeteners during your fast.

Fasting entails avoiding calorie-dense foods and liquids. Does this imply you can have a calorie-free diet soda? This is a common question among newcomers to intermittent fasting. During a fast, it is generally advised to avoid artificial sweeteners and diet drinks.

Artificial sweeteners, according to studies, can make you feel hungrier and cause you to eat more. In general, there is a lot of conflicting information and studies on artificial sweeteners and their effects on health, insulin response, blood sugar levels, and gut microbes. As a result, it's best to stick to tried-and-true intermittent fasting beverages like water, basic tea, and black coffee.

## Forget "you can't eat anything and still lose weight while intermittent fasting."

Still have questions about why you should reevaluate your diet when fasting intermittently? While consuming the same quantity of calories in a short period of time is theoretically more difficult, it is nevertheless achievable. You may be consuming a lot of calories if your food is high in saturated fat from oils, fast food, red meat, or empty calories. Furthermore, these will not be meals that are high in nutrients such as vitamins, minerals, fiber, and antioxidants. A balanced diet is therefore essential for long-term weight loss that is also excellent for the body.

## Be stressed out.

Keep your cool and remain calm. Stress might cause your cholesterol levels to rise. Fasting is not recommended if it raises stress levels in the body. Yoga and deep breathing are effective stress-relieving techniques.

## Eat too little during the eating window.

What's going on here? Yes, not eating enough is a legitimate cause of weight gain, as we have covered earlier in this chapter. However, not consuming enough food cannibalizes your muscle mass, triggering your digestion to stop, in addition to setting you up to consume too much of less-healthy items during your meal hours. You might be harming your ability to burn fat in the future if you don't build up that metabolic muscle mass.

The problem with intermittent fasting is that it's really difficult to determine your true needs because you eat according to some arbitrary time-based guidelines rather than listening to your body's indications. If you're thinking about trying an intermittent fasting diet, it's a good idea to talk to a trained dietician first to be sure you're assessing and meeting your nutritional needs properly.

**Make wrong food selections.**

We've already established that intermittent fasting focuses on the *when* rather than the *what* when it comes to eating. While this still allows you to sample a wide range of meals, it does not imply that you are free to eat whatever you want. If we're left to our own devices, most of us will choose sweet and fatty foods because they appeal to our taste buds. Pizza, cake, cookies, candy, ice cream, and processed meats, are just a few of such foods. However, this is a rather short-sighted approach. Breaking your fast with these foods will simply negate the fast's benefits.

Choose healthful, whole foods that will provide your body with all of the nutrients it requires. Vegetables, protein, healthy fats, and complex carbs should all be included in your meal. You may have heard that intermittent fasting and a low-carb diet go well together. Yes, but this is a low-carb, not a no-carb, diet. Some people try to lose weight faster by cutting out all carbs. Remember that carbohydrates provide us with calories to fuel our bodies. On your plate, include a portion of nutritious starch, preferably brown unprocessed choices.

Why should you be concerned with what you eat, when intermittent fasting is concerned with when you eat? Healthy nutrition is important for everyone, even if you aren't on a fasting regimen. You eat healthy meals since they are good for your body and keep ailments at bay. Healthy eating should be normal eating, thus we can agree that fasting should be accompanied by normal eating in this circumstance.

# 5

# EMBRACING THE LIFESTYLE

## 1. INTERMITTENT FASTING ISN'T A FAD DIET; IT'S A HEALTHY WAY OF LIFE

When the ordinary person learns about intermittent fasting for the first time, they usually remark, "Oh, I've done that before, right? You mean starving yourself to lose weight?" They're mistaken! Irregular fasting is a way of life. It's a manner of life you could live for the rest of your days.

Weight loss, enhanced mental and physical health, and other benefits are all side effects. Intermittent fasting hasn't had any negative effects on my health so far. In fact, it has greatly improved my health over time.

## 2. LISTEN TO YOUR BODY WHEN IT COMES TO DECIDING WHAT TO EAT

The intermittent fasting diet plan is one of the most often asked questions when it comes to fasting. However, as previously stated, this is not a diet plan; rather, it is an eating pattern and a way of life.

You can eat any mix of nutritious meals within the eating window. The most essential thing about what to eat is to pay attention to your body and eat accordingly. If you're fatigued and drained after eating rice or grains, for example, you might eat more veggies instead. If you feel more invigorated as a result of doing this, it's your body's way of urging you to eat more vegetables and avoid high-carb foods.

As we get older, our bodies change, and eating the same meals every day raises the risk of acquiring food intolerance and diseases. Thankfully, there is a concept of "eating by listening to your body," as described by Paul Chek, an internationally acclaimed holistic health expert, in his book How to Eat, Move and Be Healthy. The most important takeaway here is to pay attention to your body and experiment with different diets in order to achieve optimal health.

## 3. IT SIMPLIFIES YOUR LIFE

I used to be fascinated with rising early to cook breakfast, preparing six meals a day, and so on before I started intermittent fasting. Even while I made some progress toward my health goals, fat loss, muscle building, and so on, I had trouble sticking to the regimen since it was monotonous. My life is much simpler these days. I consume one or two main meals each day, don't worry over what I eat, and continue to develop my strength and health on a daily basis.

## 4. AFTER A YEAR OR SO, YOU MIGHT EXPECT YOUR RESULTS TO SLOW DOWN

I shed a lot of weight and came into the greatest shape of my life during my first year of intermittent fasting. However, after the first year, my weight and fat reduction decreased to the point where I didn't notice much of a difference.

This makes sense, because your body can only lose so much fat before it becomes harmful to your health. Simplifying my life in this way has allowed me to devote more time and energy to the things that truly matter to me.

## 5. FAST FAT REDUCTION IS ACHIEVED BY COMBINING INTERMITTENT FASTING WITH HIGH-INTENSITY INTERVAL TRAINING

If you want to reduce weight as rapidly as possible, I recommend incorporating any high-intensity training. When I originally started intermittent fasting, I added ten minutes of running three times a week, as well as weekly football matches. You could do anything you want: swimming, skipping, and jogging are all good options, and you can gradually increase the intensity until you're exhausted after each activity. Fasting helps you consume fewer calories while high-intensity workouts help you burn more calories. Your daily calorie consumption decreases dramatically, and you shed more fat over time. Simple.

## 6. INTERMITTENT FASTING CAN HELP YOU FOCUS, BE MORE PRODUCTIVE, AND BE MORE DISCIPLINED

I get a lot more work done during my fasting window, which runs from 7 a.m. to 1 p.m. on most days, than if I ate breakfast first thing in the morning. My energy levels plummet, I lose focus, and I become drowsy after I break my fast with the first meal.

As a result, before I break my fast, I've scheduled my most crucial tasks. As a result, I'm able to match my peak energy levels to my major objectives, which leads to enhanced productivity. Another thing I've seen is that the discipline of fasting every day has helped me to be more disciplined in other areas of my life. Once I began intermittent fasting, I had the strength to start a new lifestyle that included reading more, eating healthier, sleeping earlier, and so on. This is how powerful a keystone behavior can be.

## 7. FASTING ON A REGULAR BASIS MIGHT AFFECT YOUR DISCIPLINE, FOCUS, AND PRODUCTIVITY

This may appear to be in opposition to the previous statement, but consider this: a hungry guy can also be grouchy. To put it another way, when you're fasting, it's easy to lose focus and become upset because you're so hungry. This is why, rather than following a strict program, it's crucial to listen to your body. Every day, I've discovered that there's a sweet spot, a window of opportunity to break your fast. You'll waste energy that could have been used to get more work done if you break your fast too soon. You'll grow frustrated and lose attention if you break your fast very late in the day. Because every day is different, it's all about experimenting.

## 8. INTERMITTENT FASTING MAY WREAK HAVOC ON YOUR DIET

Following up on the previous point, it's easy to consume harmful or nutrient-deficient foods when you're truly hungry and break your fast. This has been one of the most difficult aspects of intermittent fasting for me.

Fasting every day requires personal discipline. Fasting and eating a healthy diet every day, however, requires superhuman discipline. The reason for this is that your body is depleted of sugar and energy while you fast. It also craves high-carbohydrate, sugary foods.

While you may be able to reach your weight-loss and appearance objectives without eating a clean diet, this may be harmful to your health in the long run. I've found that creating a successful environment and drinking as much water as possible during the day is the greatest approach to avoid this overeating inclination after breaking the fast.

## 9. INTERMITTENT FASTING HAS BEEN LINKED TO MUSCLE LOSS OR INCREASE

I damaged my lower back doing back squats during my second year of intermittent fasting and was warned to avoid lifting weights indefinitely. I was already in excellent form and assumed that things would continue to be the same. As a result,

I switched to pilates and stretching exercises in place of weight training. In addition, I began a body detox program that required me to exclude high-carb items from my diet for a few months.

My muscular mass had considerably decreased within a few weeks, to the point that my clothes no longer fit as well. My daily calorie intake was substantially lowered as a result of the detox program and intermittent fasting strategy, which contributed to muscle loss. I resumed my weight-training regimen and increased my carb intake after my recovery, while maintaining my intermittent fasting strategy. I restored my physical shape and gained back the muscle that I had lost after only a few months. The main takeaway is that calorie intake is really important.

## 10. BECAUSE IT ALLOWS YOU TO CONSUME FEWER CALORIES, INTERMITTENT FASTING IS EFFECTIVE.

I thought I had discovered the golden formula to weight loss and healthy life during my first year of intermittent fasting, just like any rookie. Because it worked so well for me, I would preach to everyone about how this was the only way to achieve their health goals. As I explored more over the years, I learned that the reason intermittent fasting is so good for weight loss is because it drives you to eat less.

The less calories you consume and the more weight you shed, the better. That's all there is to it. It's not a trick of the light. Some people who try intermittent fasting regard it as a waste of time since it doesn't work for them. However, in the vast majority of cases, they failed to keep track of their calorie consumption.

Intermittent fasting is just another way to help you cut down on your calorie intake. However, if you choose to devour junk food every day after your fast, you may end up gaining more weight than before! In other words, as I've already stated, the number of calories you consume each day is quite important. Intermittent fasting should not be used as an excuse to eat too much ice cream or lose track of your good eating habits. This is why eating six or more meals per day could help you attain your health goals. You'll lose weight over time if the total calories you consume each day are less than the calories you expend to move and live.

## 11. ALLOWING YOURSELF TO FAST INTERMITTENTLY SHOULD NOT KEEP YOU FROM LIVING YOUR LIFE

The most important thing I've learned during my four years of intermittent fasting is to quit stressing about being perfect and just live your life. I refused to break my fast outside of my eating window during my first year. I'd go on vacation to new places, bypassing the opportunity to eat new foods from diverse cultures because I was fasting.

I used to be extremely set in my ways when it came to intermittent fasting. But, as time has passed, I've come to realize that there's more to life than meeting my exercise, nutrition, and fitness goals. I continue to work toward my health objectives every week, but I don't punish myself if I don't meet them. Instead of fasting, I occasionally have a meal for breakfast. I occasionally break my fast at the appropriate time, but then eat unhealthy meals.

## LET'S GET STARTED: THE STEPS

It's important to note that intermittent fasting is not a diet. It is a method of eating that is timed. Intermittent fasting, unlike a dietary plan that restricts where calories originate from, does not define which items a person should eat or avoid. Although intermittent fasting has various health benefits, including weight loss, it is not for everyone.

Intermittent fasting entails alternating between eating and fasting times. People may find it challenging at first to eat only for a short period of time each day or to alternate between eating and not eating days. This book includes advice on how to get started fasting, such as setting personal goals, preparing meals, and determining caloric requirements. Intermittent fasting is a common way for people to:

- Simplify their lives.
- Lose some weight.
- Improve their general health and well-being, such as slowing down the aging process.

Fasting is generally safe for most healthy, well-nourished people, however it may not be acceptable for those with medical issues. The following guidelines are intended to assist individuals who are ready to begin fasting in making it as simple and successful as possible.

**1. Get clear on your goals.**

Clear goals will help you get a long way in life, but don't overlook the necessity of setting your goals before beginning an intermittent fasting practice.

It was shedding the additional weight I had gained during and after pregnancy (which cured a slew of other health issues for me), that increased my metabolic health and allowed me to obtain more mental clarity and focus. In general, I wanted to be in better health for my own benefit and, most significantly, for the sake of my child. However, my research revealed that in order to fully profit from intermittent fasting, I needed to clarify exactly what I desired from it. And allow me to explain why this is so.

For a variety of reasons, defining your goals when it comes to intermittent fasting is crucial. First and foremost, it enables you to select the most appropriate intermittent fasting approach to get you closer to your goals. The alternate-day intermittent fasting approach, for example, is better for weight loss, whereas the 16/8 method is more of a good lifestyle adjustment.

While weight loss is one of the most common reasons individuals try intermittent fasting, you may have your own motivations for giving it a try. Determine what you want to get out of the diet before moving on to the next step.

**2. Choose an intermittent fasting method.**

Now that you know what you want to get out of intermittent fasting, the following step is to choose an intermittent fasting approach that will help you reach your objectives. Other considerations, in addition to your specific goals for intermittent fasting, play a role in selecting an intermittent fasting approach that will provide you with the most benefits. To mention a few, these factors include how long you want to fast, your daily routine, what field you work in, what a typical workday looks like for you, the climatic conditions in your area of the world, and how often you dine out with friends and family.

However, once you've decided on an intermittent fasting approach, keep in mind that you're not committed to it indefinitely. If you find that your current intermittent fasting regimen isn't working for you, or if you think you've mastered the moderate forms of intermittent fasting (think of the 16/8 method) and want to go pro and explore some more challenging routes, such as alternate-day fasting, it's completely possible. Furthermore, it is recommended that a person give any intermittent fasting approach at least one month of careful consideration before quitting or switching it up for good.

**3. Calculate your calorie requirements.**

The next stage is to calculate and balance your calorie intake so you know what you want to get out of intermittent fasting and how you'll go about doing it. This is significant because, if your primary aim for intermittent fasting is weight loss, you must consume fewer calories than you expend for energy, resulting in a calorie deficit. While intermittent fasting is supposed to create a calorie deficit while you're fasting, if you're not careful with the calories you consume during your eating windows, it can soon turn into a surplus.

People who practice intermittent fasting are usually the least concerned with calorie counting and measurement. Although keeping track of one's calorie consumption is important to some extent (even when fasting intermittently), some people believe that their calorie consumption is taken care of automatically as a result of fasting intermittently. While this may be beneficial for people who don't have (or aren't at risk for) eating disorders like anorexia and binge eating, it might be harmful for people who have eating disorders that are exacerbated by intermittent fasting.

It's also vital to keep track of how many calories you take in during intermittent fasting since, while some types of intermittent fasting, such as alternate-day fasting, allow for calorie consumption on fasting days, there's a limit to how many calories you can ingest. This restriction is in place to make the benefits of intermittent fasting, such as weight loss, more accessible.

Furthermore, there is a prevalent belief that if you consume less than fifty calories in the morning, you would be deemed to be fasting. This is especially important for people who follow the 16/8 technique, which involves eating a late dinner and a later breakfast in order to fast for sixteen hours. These people can consume plain water or a cup of black coffee (with no added sugar) in the mornings without breaking their fast.

But, guess what? This also means that you must be conscious of the calories you ingest in order to avoid sabotaging your intermittent fasting practice. All of this points to one conclusion: in order to reach your intermittent fasting goals, you must keep track of your calorie consumption, whether you're fasting or feasting. At the very least, at first.

Today, there are a variety of programs that may be used to track calorie consumption. "MyFitnessPal" and "Lose It," which feature a calorie counter as well as a food diary and an exercise log, are two of the best.

The focus on calorie intake will normally fade into the background as intermittent fasting and your new eating habits get established in your schedule as you get the hang of it in whichever method or shape you think best suits you. Because you know the approximate amount you consume daily, you will find that you don't need to watch calories as much. This is when the much-touted benefit of not having to calculate calories reappears, kicking and screaming! Your daily caloric intake is more or less at your fingertips now that you've had more practice and have built a good pattern and habit of following your intermittent fasting lifestyle. As a result, you don't have to worry about it as much because you can go about your everyday activities without worrying about your calorie intake.

**4. Create a meal plan.**

Also, no. I'm not going to contradict myself right now. Intermittent fasting is freeing in the sense that it allows you to avoid having to schedule meals all of the time. And I'm not going back on my previous statements. This is a completely optional step. You have the option of doing or not doing it. Intermittent fasting is not a dietary limitation.

Regardless of whether you practice intermittent fasting or not, we all know that a well-balanced and nutritious diet is essential for optimum health. One thing to keep in mind is that depriving yourself of meals for a specific amount of time does not excuse you from eating junk food when your eating window eventually opens. When you finally sit down to eat after an intermittent fasting program, making improper food choices is not only bad for your overall health, but it also squanders all of your intermittent fasting efforts. And you don't want that to happen.

As a result, it's a good idea to set aside some time to (informally) plan your weekly meals. This will not only help you keep track of your calorie consumption (and thus regularly lose and maintain weight), but it will also ensure that you have everything you need to prepare a healthy, nutritious, and enjoyable dinner. Because, let's face it, when preparing a nutritious meal at home becomes tough for whatever reason, we're more likely to order takeout and consume unhealthy snacks. And, to be honest, if you're consuming a lot of bad food when you're not fasting, you might as well not fast at all!

## 5. Calculate body mass index.

The body mass index, or BMI, is a measurement of how healthy your current weight is in relation to your height. Your BMI is calculated by multiplying your weight in kilograms by your height in square meters. You are healthy if your values are between 18.5 and 24.9. Anything under 18.5 is unhealthy. Women should have a measurement of 21 and men should have a measurement of 23. This figure, however, does not take into account body fat, waist circumference, eating habits, or lifestyle. All of these contribute to your overall wellness.

If you're a man, your BMI may be greater, but it doesn't imply you should reduce weight if you're healthy. If your BMI is greater than 30, you are considered obese. However, this isn't limited to the number because a good weight can be accompanied by an excessive quantity of body fat. These are basic estimations that may lead you to consider someone athletic as well as someone who is slimmer but has a high body fat percentage as obese. In consultation with your doctor and a dietician, measuring your BMI can help you define your weight loss objectives.

**6. Consult with your doctor.**

You should discuss with your doctor about your food plans once you've decided on an intermittent fasting style and strategy. Based on your medical history and current health conditions, if any, your doctor can advise you. Throughout your intermittent fasting adventure, keep these tips in mind, make sure to seek medical guidance to ensure you're not jeopardizing your health. The goal is to lose weight in a healthy and long-term manner.

**7. Prepare your mind.**

Intermittent fasting can be physically and mentally demanding. You can have days when you feel defeated because you didn't stick to your diet plan to the letter. When you don't see any visible changes in your weight, you may become discouraged.

Keep in mind that intermittent fasting is a journey that takes time to complete and requires ongoing mental renewal. To stay dedicated to the process, make sure you're in a healthy mental state before you start.

## 8. Remove toxins.

Getting rid of toxins in your body is a fantastic approach to prepare for intermittent fasting. This includes limiting alcohol, caffeine, and refined sugar consumption. These meals cause you to retain water, causing you to feel bloated and sluggish. During this process, you will require as much natural energy as possible.

## CONCLUSION

To ensure a good journey, you must take some actions to prepare for intermittent fasting. Don't decide to perform intermittent fasting on a spur of the moment. You must educate yourself on the many types of intermittent fasting, consult your doctor, and mentally and physically prepare yourself.

Remember that everyone's path with intermittent fasting is different. Once you've made the decision to begin, look for social networking groups that include members that are on the same weight-loss path as you. After all, inspiration and support can help you get through the procedure more quickly. You can also use apps made specifically for intermittent fasting.

# 6

# COMBINE INTERMITTENT FASTING WITH HEALTHY HABITS

Are you considering increasing your physical activity? Have you been attempting to reduce your consumption of less nutritious foods? Are you attempting to eat healthier and move more, but finding it difficult to maintain these changes?

Old habits are difficult to break. Changing your habits is a multistep process. It can take some time for adjustments to become new habits. You might also come across obstructions along the path.

Embracing a new, better lifestyle might help you prevent serious health problems like diabetes and obesity. Two new habits that may aid in weight loss and increased vigor are a healthy diet and frequent physical activity. If you keep to these guidelines, you'll be fine. Modifications will last for a while, so it's possible that they'll get ingrained in your daily habit.

When it comes to modifying your health habits or behavior, there are four steps to consider. You'll also get advice on how to enhance your food habits, physical activity levels, and overall health. There are five steps to improving one's health behavior:

1. Precontemplation
2. Contemplation
3. Preparation
4. Action
5. Maintenance

What level of transformation are you in?

## PRECONTEMPLATION

You don't realize there's an issue at this point, and you have no intention of changing. "I'm simply unwinding after a day of work. There's nothing wrong with a couple drinks at the end of the day!" a person who drinks more than two alcoholic beverages per day might argue.

## CONTEMPLATION: "I'M THINKING ABOUT IT."

You're thinking about change and getting excited to get started in this first stage. If you're reading this, you might be in this stage. Here are some other signs of being in the contemplation stage:

- You have been thinking about making a change but aren't quite ready to do so.
- You feel that forming new habits will improve your health, energy level, or general well-being.
- You're unsure how you'll get beyond the obstacles that are preventing you from making a change.

## PREPARATION: "I'VE MADE UP MY MIND TO DO SOMETHING."

You are now in the planning stage, and you are considering particular concepts that will work for you. You might be in this phase if:

- You have made the decision to change and are prepared to take action.
- You have set some precise objectives that you'd like to achieve.
- You are preparing to put your strategy into action.

## ACTON: "I'VE BEGUN TO MAKE CHANGES."

You're in the third stage now, and you're putting your plan into action and achieving the goals you set earlier. You may well be in this stage if:

- You have made changes in nutrition and physical

exercise in the last five months or so, as well as other behavior changes.

- You are getting used to how it feels to eat more nutritiously, be more energetic, and make other lifestyle adjustments like getting more sleep or limiting screen time.
- You've been attempting to overcome obstacles to your achievement.

## MAINTENANCE: "I'VE ADOPTED A NEW ROUTINE."

You've become used to your alterations and have kept them up for more than six months at this point. You may well be in this stage if:

- Your adjustments have become second nature to you.
- You've come up with inventive strategies to stick to your schedule.
- You've experienced setbacks and blunders, but you've been able to overcome them and continue moving forward.

## IS IT BETTER TO DEVELOP HEALTHY HABITS ALONE OR WITH THE HELP OF A SUPPORT GROUP?

Healthy behaviors are contagious, it turns out! When one spouse in a couple makes a healthy lifestyle adjustment (such as stopping smoking, exercising, or losing weight), their partner is significantly more likely to follow suit. Similarly, having healthier friends or people in your social network will often push you to make healthier choices as well.

It's great if you're internally driven to get started with long-term improvement. However, if you have that inner urge to make a change, having a support group may be quite beneficial in taking you through the five stages outlined above in a healthy manner. You can learn about other people's challenges, accomplishments, and failures, which can help you prepare for your own. Weight loss, addiction treatment, and a variety of other lifestyle changes have all been demonstrated to benefit from having a social support group.

## WHAT ARE THE ADVANTAGES OF HAVING A HEALTHY EATING SUPPORT SYSTEM?

Having a support system can help you on your health journey in a variety of ways, both major and small. Here are some of the ways that having a support system can help you:

- **Emotional assistance:** When things get tough, encouragement from loved ones can keep you going.
- **Helpful suggestions:** Tips from people who are on the same path as you might show you how to make a practical change to a healthy lifestyle.
- **Developing a culture of accountability:** Knowing that you'll be sharing your progress with others once a week will help you stay motivated to achieve your goals.
- **Setting a good example:** Seeing someone else successfully quit smoking or reduce weight might inspire you and show you how to reach your own goals.

## IS IT TRUE THAT HAVING A SUPPORT SYSTEM CAN HELP YOU ACHIEVE YOUR WEIGHT-LOSS GOALS?

Yes. Having a support system boosts your chances of achieving your weight-loss objectives. If you're not sure where to start looking for help, try these options:

- **Join an organization that already has a support structure in place:** Weight Watchers is an example of this.
- **Look for local organizations that already exist:** This can take the form of online support groups

like Facebook groups or in-person neighborhood groups like a local meetup group for people who wish to go for walks together.
- **Form your own support system:** Friends, relatives, coworkers, members of your religious group, and other connections may be able to assist you. They can help you form a social support network to assist you in your weight-loss efforts.

## WHAT SMALL, HEALTHY IMPROVEMENTS CAN I MAKE AT HOME TODAY?

Starting small is the best way to make long-term changes. Concentrate on specific examples that have a distinct action, frequency, and duration. It's simpler to adopt new healthy behaviors once you've established tiny routines that have become habitual. Simple and useful goal examples vary depending on which aspect of your life you want to focus on initially.

### Diet

If you want to eat healthier foods or lose weight, you can work on:

- Consuming at least five fruits and vegetables per day. As needed, change your goal: If you don't eat any fruits or veggies now, setting a target of one to two fruits

and vegetables per day can be enough to get you started.
- Using whole-grain bread instead of white bread.
- Limiting red meat consumption to once per week (or once a month).
- Swapping sugary drinks for water with a few slices of fruit for added flavor.
- Drinking six to eight cups of water every day as recommended.

## Exercise

If you want to increase your physical activity, you could try:

- Every morning, go for a twenty-minute stroll.
- At work, instead of taking the elevator, take the stairs.
- Instead of a weekly happy hour, ask a friend to join you for a weekly walk.
- Attend a yoga or dance class on a weekly basis.
- Participate in a local sports league.

## Mental health

If you wish to improve your mental health, you could try:

- Getting a meditation app and committing to five minutes of meditation every day.
- Working on your deep breathing methods.

- Writing for ten minutes each day in a journal.
- Keeping a gratitude jar in your kitchen and jotting down three things you're grateful for every day.
- Volunteering—it's been proven that helping others is good for your mental health.

## Sleep

If you wish to improve your sleep, you can do the following:

- Get an old-fashioned alarm clock and keep your phone in a different room at night so it doesn't distract you before bed or while you're sleeping.
- Make a vow to exclusively use your bed for sleep and sex. Your body will develop a strong association between the bed and sleep over time, making it easier for you to fall asleep.
- Determine what bedtime will provide you with seven to eight hours of sleep each night, and stick to it every night.
- Take a break from screens for thirty minutes before going to bed.
- In the afternoon and evening, limit your intake of alcohol and caffeine.

## The bottom line

It is difficult, but not impossible, to change your behaviors. Always remember to start small. It's a lot more difficult to "start eating healthier" than it is to "eat five fruits and veggies every day." You can improve your chances of success in developing a healthy lifestyle by mentally preparing ahead of time and finding a support network.

## HEALTHY HABITS

The majority of us aspire to live long, happy, prosperous, and healthy lives. Unfortunately, in our quest for achievement, we frequently sacrifice our health, and as a result, we end up with a variety of maladies and disabilities that we could have prevented.

That does not have to be the case. Despite the fact that many of us lead stressful, demanding lives, we can build habits that will help us live healthier and more productive lives with a little adjusting here and there.

There's no shortage of advice on how to live a healthy lifestyle—one book I saw recommended 107 beneficial habits! I won't go into detail, but I've identified the most common nineteen healthy behaviors that anyone should be able to incorporate into their daily routine.

## 1. Get your exercise.

"Those who exercised four days per week were less likely than sedentary persons to develop diabetes, heart disease, and high cholesterol," according to one study. Adults should acquire 150 minutes of moderate aerobic activity per week, according to the American Heart Association, to maintain their heart and blood vessels' health. That works out to about thirty minutes per day, five days a week. Many folks require more physical activity than necessary to lose weight. Strength training two to three times per week also aids in the maintenance of strong bones and muscles.

Because physical activity is vital for overall health, it's better to pick an activity that you enjoy so that getting your 150 minutes in each week is a pleasure rather than a job. Walking is a great, low-cost, go-anywhere activity, but there are a plethora of other ways to stay active. If you despise going to the gym, try watching fitness videos on your computer or iPad from the comfort of your own home. If you prefer to exercise in a group, there are a variety of fitness courses available, ranging from indoor cycling to yoga. There are numerous ways to stay active, including boxing, inline skating, and rowing to relieve tension. Find something exciting to keep you from being bored, burned out, or giving up. It's also fine to do brief bursts of exercise rather than thirty minutes or more at a time.

## 2. Don't skip breakfast.

Breakfast eaters consume more vitamins and minerals while consuming less fat and cholesterol, according to research. Consuming foods with lots of fiber and protein will keep you feeling full and energized. Low-fat milk, fruit, yogurt, as well as whole-grain cereals and breads, are all examples of these healthy foods.

## 3. Maintain a healthy eating routine throughout the day.

Consuming more fruit and nuts, as well as avoiding sugary drinks and snacks, are examples of this behavior. The American Heart Association suggests eating fish twice a week at mealtime. Fatty fish (tuna, herring, salmon, mackerel, lake trout, and sardines) are high in omega-3 fatty acids, which help to lower the risk of heart disease.

Remember to keep note of your servings. If you want to live to be a hundred, eat more fruits and vegetables high in vitamins, minerals, and fiber, and eat less high-calorie items high in sugar and fats.

And remember to chew your meal! To acquire the most digestible form, many nutritionists advocate chewing each mouthful twenty to thirty times. Chewing slowly also reduces calorie intake by around 10 percent, according to studies, partially because it takes your stomach about twenty minutes to signal your brain that it's full.

Finally, a word of caution about a healthy eating habit: synthesized sweeteners should be avoided. Artificial sweeteners may be linked to an increased risk of high blood pressure, diabetes, weight gain, obesity, and heart disease, according to a ten-year study published in the Canadian Medical Association Journal by Gold Bee researchers. "Most patients who consume artificial sweeteners do so in the expectation that these products will help them prevent weight gain, diabetes, and heart disease," said Dr. Meghan Azad, chief author of the CMAJ research. Many other studies, however, show the inverse relationship.

## 4. Keep yourself hydrated.

Every single cell, tissue, and organ in the body requires water, therefore getting the correct amount is critical. We've been taught for generations that our bodies require an eight-ounce glass of water per day, a quantity that has never been scientifically validated. Perhaps a better metric is to drink enough water to urinate once every two to four hours and have light-colored urine. Many technologies, ranging from "smart bottles" to countless free applications, are easily available to help you start and maintain this habit.

## 5. Challenge yourself.

We all get trapped in ruts, doing the same things over and over again, but taking on challenges keeps your body and mind flexible. Also, don't be embarrassed if you're not an expert. Keep in mind that every expert was once a novice.

## 6. Don't neglect dental hygiene.

How many people floss their teeth at the conclusion of a long day? According to some research, flossing on a regular basis can add up to six years to your life. Why? According to this notion, bacteria that cause plaque enters the mouth's bloodstream and are connected to inflammation, which leads to clogging of arteries and heart disease. Make flossing your teeth a habit before going to bed, and you'll live longer.

## 7. Learn something new.

Learning new abilities is beneficial to your mental health. Enroll in a dance class or a session on creative writing. Even better, learn a new language. The mental effort required by these new activities can help to decrease the aging process and potentially delay the onset of Alzheimer's disease.

## 8. Go offline.

Do you spend a lot of time checking your email and social media? Sure, you may see your friends' and family's most recent updates with a single click, but do you really need to see photos of your cousin's most recent meal? Allow it to wait until the morning. Make a schedule for when you'll log off and put down the phone. When you reduce your screen time, you have more time to accomplish something else. Go for a walk, read a book, or assist your cousin in chopping vegetables for their next delicious meal.

## 9. Get rid of the pessimists.

Whether you're on a new diet or passionate about something, it's critical to say the right things to the appropriate people. Whether you have a lot of negative individuals in your life or you know someone who does, don't bring them along on your new adventure. It's critical to have the right support system in place when starting a new diet or lifestyle. Others will need to help you succeed by assisting you, inspiring you, and supporting your new route.

## 10. Don't smoke.

According to studies, non-smokers have a substantially lower probability of developing chronic health problems. Smoking was found to be a very strong risk factor for strokes and death.

Smoking causes or exacerbates a slew of health issues, including diabetes, heart disease, and many other less well-known issues. Quitting cigarettes hastily improves your health; the first signs (a decreased heart rate and blood pressure) appear within twenty minutes after your last puff. According to Lisa Connor, a smoke-free lifestyle and a nutritious diet can result in a seven-year difference in lifespan compared to people who smoke.

Even if you've previously tried to quit smoking but failed, Connor advises, "Don't give up trying!" Most smokers attempt to quit several times before finally succeeding. While some people quit smoking cold turkey, research shows that using nicotine replacement products (such as nicotine gum or the skin patch) or prescription medicine, as well as joining a support group, are the most effective techniques for quitting smoking.

## 11. Train your muscles.

Strength training aids in the conversion of fat to muscle mass. As a result, even if you're a couch potato, you'll burn more calories. These routines, on the other hand, can help you lose weight, strengthen your heart, and strengthen your bones. At least twice a week, do strength-training exercises including push-ups, lunges, and weight lifting.

## 12. Head outdoors.

One of the simplest methods to boost your general health is to get some fresh air on a daily basis. Vitamin D is produced by the body when it is exposed to the sun, and it has been demonstrated to have several important activities in the body. Vitamin-D deficiency has been related to weariness, a reduced immune system, bone and back pain, as well as melancholy and low mood. Vitamin D is one of the most widely supplemented vitamins, despite the fact that daily sun exposure may be a simple solution to this problem. So, whether it's spring, summer, winter, or fall, make it a point to get outside every day.

## 13. Go to bed early.

The only time during the day when our bodies can relax, unwind, and rejuvenate is when we sleep. Unfortunately, many people do not get the recommended eight hours of sleep per night, which can have serious health consequences. Many people put off going to bed in favor of other activities such as television, social media, and video games, but this can harm our health over time. Sleep deprivation, or sleep of low quality, has been related to memory problems, mood swings, decreased immunity, changing eating habits, and premature aging. Additionally, hormone abnormalities in insulin, leptin, cortisol, and a range of other hormones have been linked to a lack of sleep, and all of these factors have an impact on weight. Furthermore, going to sleep in a timely fashion makes it simpler to get up early in the morning, this is among the most crucial healthy daily habits you can develop. So, if you're a night owl, set a curfew for yourself to get to bed a little earlier since, let's face it, nothing constructive happens after 10:00 p.m. Turn off all electronic gadgets, dim the lights, read a book, and concentrate on getting a good night's sleep.

## 14. Wake up early.

You don't have to get up with the sun every day, but waking up at a sensible (early) hour is essential for optimum health. The human body and brain have evolved to follow a twenty-four-hour clock that helps with sleep. In the regulation of sleep and waking patterns dictated by our natural surroundings, notably the rising and setting of the sun. Cortisol levels, a hormone known for its role in immunity, metabolism and stress response, are also linked to the circadian tempo and energy degree. Cortisol levels begin to rise two to three hours after the onset of sleep in a balanced condition and continue to rise until the early morning, assisting us in waking up. Cortisol levels in the body will then reach a peak about 8:30 or 9:00 a.m. and then progressively fall during the day. Following the body's natural circadian tempo and cortisol levels, on the contrary, is an easy method to lift vigor, efficiency, and general well-being.

## 15. Stop weighing yourself.

This relates to my previous remarks on calories. Some people are obsessed with their weight. Every morning and night, they weigh themselves. They are thrilled if they lose weight. However, if they gain weight, they are more likely to get depressed. Please don't get me wrong: you should surely strive for a healthy weight. This, on the other hand, will be a natural result of eating well and exercising consistently.

## 16. Consider a more positive perspective.

A negative attitude leads to a negative life. If you're one of those people who always sees the glass as half empty, consider why you think that way. It could just be a result of beliefs you've acquired, but remember that you always have a choice in how you perceive things. Next time, explore an alternative, more optimistic viewpoint. If you do this on a regular basis, you will notice a gradual shift in your perspective on the world.

## 17. Eat more greens.

Vegetables are high in vitamins, minerals, and fiber, which may help maintain a balanced stomach, prevent constipation, and other digestive difficulties. More than three servings of veggies per day reduced the risk of coronary heart disease and stroke by about 20 percent compared to individuals who ate less than three servings per day. In addition, incorporating more veggies into your diet reduces your intake of processed foods, refined carbohydrates, and added sugars.

## 18. Maintain your balance.

Good balance will help you avoid injuries if you're young and active. If you're older, it will keep you active for longer and reduce your chances of breaking a bone if you fall. Balance, regardless of age, means stronger muscle tone, a healthier heart, and more self-assurance. Yoga and tai chi are excellent ways to improve it, but any activity that keeps you moving, even walking, will do you good.

## 19. Be mindful.

It might be as simple as meditating or simply taking a moment to smell the blossoms. Mindfulness reduces stress, relieves pain, and enhances your mood, according to studies. And scientists are starting to figure out how. According to one study, eight weeks of consistent meditation can alter areas of the brain associated with emotions, learning, and memory. Even doing the dishes can be beneficial to your brain if done thoughtfully.

## BREAKFAST RECIPES

If you completely neglect fats and don't consider the macronutrients you're putting into your system, it's possible to wind up eating too many calories or not getting adequate fats, proteins, or carbs to effectively energize your body.

Are you ready to start an intermittent fasting diet? Here's a plan you can use to make sure your meals keep you energized and the fasting period goes by quickly. You'll be an intermittent fasting pro if you combine these recipes to create your own unique meal plan.

## 1. SWEET POTATOES WITH EGG SCRAMBLE

Total time: 25 minutes

Servings: 1

**Ingredients:**

- 1 sweet potato, diced (8 oz.)
- ½ cup onion, chopped
- 2 teaspoons rosemary, sliced
- Salt and pepper
- 4 big eggs
- 4 big egg whites
- 2 tablespoons chive, minced

**Directions:**

1. Warm up the oven to 425 degrees (F). Toss the rosemary, onion, sweet potato, and salt and pepper on a baking sheet. Spray with cooking spray and cook until soft, about 20 minutes.
2. Meanwhile, whisk together the eggs, egg whites, and a pinch of salt and pepper in a medium mixing bowl. Scramble the eggs in a skillet sprayed with cooking spray for about 5 minutes on medium.
3. Serve with the spuds and a sprinkling of minced chives.

Per serving: 20g fat, 44g protein, 571 calories, 52g carbs (9g fiber).

## 2. TURMERIC TOFU SCRAMBLES

Total time: 15 minutes

Servings: 1

**Ingredients:**

- 1 Portobello mushroom
- three or four cherry tomatoes
- 1 tablespoon olive oil, with a little extra for brushing
- Salt and pepper
- ½ pound (14 oz.) firm tofu
- ¼ teaspoon turmeric powder
- 1 teaspoon garlic powder
- ½ cup avocado, thinly sliced

**Directions:**

1. Preheat the oven to 400 degrees (F). Brush the mushrooms and tomatoes with oil and arrange them on a baking sheet. Salt and pepper to taste. Roast for about 10 minutes, or until the vegetables are soft.
2. Meanwhile, add the tofu, turmeric, garlic powder, and a pinch of salt in a medium mixing bowl. Using a fork,

mash the potatoes. Heat 1 tablespoon olive oil in a large skillet over medium heat. Cook, stirring regularly, until the tofu mixture is firm and egg-like, about 3 minutes.

3. Serve the tofu with the mushroom, tomatoes, and avocado on a plate.

Per serving: 431 calories, 21g protein, 17g carbs (8g fiber), 33g fat.

## 3. AVOCADO RICOTTA POWER TOAST

Total time: 5 minutes

Servings: 1

### Ingredients:

- 1 whole-grain bread slice
- ¼ cup avocados, smashed
- 2 tablespoons ricotta
- a pinch of crushed red pepper flakes
- a pinch of flaky salt

### Directions:

1. Toast the bread and spread avocado, ricotta, crushed red pepper flakes, and sea salt on top. Serve with

scrambled or hard-boiled eggs with yogurt or fruit on the side.

Per serving: 288 calories, 10g protein, 29g carbs (10g fiber), 17g fat.

## 4. ALMOND APPLE SPICE MUFFINS

Total time: 15 minutes

Servings: 5

**Ingredients:**

- ½ pound butter
- 2 cups almond flour
- 4 spoonfuls vanilla protein powder
- 4 big eggs
- 1 cup applesauce, unsweetened
- 1 tablespoon cinnamon powder
- 1 tablespoon allspice
- 1 teaspoon cloves
- 2 tablespoons baking powder

## Directions:

1. Preheat the oven to 350° (F). Melt the butter in a small microwave-safe bowl on low power for about 30 seconds.
2. Combine all of the remaining ingredients with the melted butter in a mixing bowl. Use cupcake liners or spray two muffin tins using nonstick cooking spray.
3. Fill the muffin tins about ¾ filled with batter, being careful not to overfill. This recipe should yield 10 muffins.
4. Bake for 12 minutes on one pan in the oven. If you overbake the muffins, they will become too dry. Remove the first pan from the oven when it's done baking and repeat with the second muffin tin.

Per serving: 484 calories, 40g protein, 16g carbs (5g fiber), 31g fat.

## 5. BOWL OF ROASTED VEGGIES AND SAVORY OATS

The new way to eat oatmeal is with savory oats! It's the ultimate nutritious comfort food in a bowl, with rich and cheesy oats topped with roasted veggies, a fried egg, and bacon.

Total time: 45 minutes

Servings: 1

## Ingredients:

- 16 oz. butternut squash, diced
- 8 oz. Brussels sprouts, halved
- 1 tablespoon extra-virgin olive oil
- 1 teaspoon salt
- 1 teaspoon black pepper
- 1 tablespoon butter
- ½ cup onion, finely chopped
- 2 cups Quaker Old Fashioned Oats
- 2 quarts water
- ½ cup shredded sharp cheddar cheese
- 4 eggs
- 2 cooked turkey bacon strips, crumbled

## Directions:

1. Preheat the oven to 400 degrees (F). Using parchment paper, line a large baking sheet.
2. Toss the Brussels sprouts, olive oil, butternut squash, chopped onion, 1/2 teaspoon salt, and 1/2 teaspoon black pepper together in a large mixing basin, then place on the baking sheet.
3. Bake for 20 to 22 minutes, or until the vegetables are golden brown and soft.
4. Melt the butter in a medium pot over medium heat

while the vegetables roast. To toast the oats, add them to the pan and cook for 30 seconds. Bring the water to a low boil, then reduce to a low heat. Reduce to a low heat and continue to cook for 8 to 10 minutes, or until the oats acquire a thick consistency, adding more water as needed. Season with the remaining salt and black pepper and stir in the shredded cheese. Keep warm.

5. Cook eggs sunny-side up or over easy in a large greased non-stick pan.
6. Fill a bowl halfway with oats, then top with veggies, an egg, and bacon crumbles.

Per serving: 19.9 protein, 56.7 carbs, 0.2g trans-fat, 7.3g saturated fat, 16.9 fat, 816.3mg sodium, 6g sugar, 460 calories.

## 6. SPINACH AND BACON MINI QUICHES

Total time: 25 minutes

Servings: 1

**Ingredients:**

- 6 eggs
- 3 tablespoons milk
- ¾ cup spinach, finely chopped
- 1 cup shredded cheddar cheese
- 4 bacon strips, cooked and sliced

- a pinch of pepper

## Directions:

1. Preheat the oven to 350 degrees (F) and butter a mini muffin pan.
2. Whisk together the eggs and milk in a large mixing dish. Combine the chopped bacon, shredded cheddar, chopped spinach, and pepper. To combine all of the ingredients, give it a brisk stir.
3. Pour the egg blend evenly into the muffin pan cups.
4. Bake in the oven for 15 to 18 minutes.
5. Allow mini quiches to cool off in the pan before carefully taking it out with a little knife after they are done.

Per serving: 53g cholesterol, 3.5g protein, 1.5g saturated fat, 3.5g fat, 82mg sodium, 470 calories.

## 7. BUDDHA BOWL

Total time: 25 minutes

Servings: 2

## Ingredients:

- 2 pastured eggs, poached

- 2 sausages (we used a spicy lamb sausage), pre-cooked
- 1 cup riced cauliflower
- grass-fed ghee for cooking
- 1 avocado, sliced
- a quarter cucumber, sliced
- 2 handfuls lightly steamed organic leafy greens
- Garnish with: a wedge of lemons, sliced spring onions, sliced chilli, fresh herbs, salt to taste

## Directions:

1. Preheat a frying pan over medium-high heat.
2. Melt 1–2 tablespoons of ghee evenly throughout the pan. Add the cauliflower rice and cook until it is done to your liking.
3. Place the leafy greens on a plate or in a big mixing basin.
4. Place the cauliflower rice beside the leafy leaves once it's ready.
5. Reheat the sausages in the same frying pan.
6. Meanwhile, arrange the avocado, cucumber slices, and poached eggs on top of the cauliflower rice and leafy greens as desired.
7. When the sausages are done, add them to the bowl with the rest of the ingredients.
8. Garnish with your garnishes, then serve and enjoy!

Per serving: 13g fat, 25gmg cholesterol, 233mg sodium, 8g fiber, 2.5g sugar, 25g protein.

## 8. BERRY MATCHA SMOOTHIE

Total time: 5 minutes

Servings: 2

### Ingredients:

- 1 quart coconut milk
- 1 cup water
- 1–1.5 cup organic frozen berries
- half an avocado
- 1 tablespoon Brain Octane C8 MCT Oil
- 1 scoop Bulletproof Vanilla Bean Collagen Protein
- 1 scoop Inner Fuel Bulletproof Prebiotic
- 1 teaspoon matcha powder
- ½–1 teaspoon vanilla extract
- (optional) ice and a sweetener of choice, to taste

### Directions:

1. In a blender, combine all of the ingredients and blend until totally smooth.
2. Taste and make any adjustments you'd like.
3. Pour into two glasses and serve right away.

Per serving: 496 calories, 40.9g fat, 56mg salt, 30g carbs, 10g fibre, 7.5g sugar, 10.7 g protein.

## 9. FETA-FILLED TOMATO-TOPPED OLDIE OMELETTE

Total time: 11 minutes

Servings: 1

**Ingredients:**

- 1 tablespoon coconut oil
- 2 eggs
- 1.5 tablespoon milk
- A dash of salt and pepper
- ¼ cup tomatoes, sliced into cubes
- 2 tablespoons feta cheese, crumbled

**Directions:**

1. Beat the eggs with pepper, salt, milk, and remaining spices.
2. Pour the mixture into a heated pan with coconut oil.
3. Stir in the tomatoes and cheese. Cook for 6 minutes or until the cheese melts.

Per serving: 335 calories, 28.4g fat, 16.2g protein, 4.5g carbs, 0.8g fiber.

## 10. CARROT BREAKFAST SALAD

Total time: 4 hours

Servings: 4

**Ingredients:**

- 2 tablespoons olive oil
- 2 lbs. baby carrots, peeled and halved
- 3 garlic cloves, minced
- 2 yellow onions, chopped
- ½ cup vegetable stock
- ⅓ cup tomatoes, crushed
- A pinch of salt and black pepper

**Directions:**

1. In your slow cooker, combine all the ingredients, cover, and cook on high for 4 hours.
2. Divide into bowls and serve for breakfast.

Per serving: 437 calories, 2.39g protein, 39.14 fat, 23.28g carbs.

## 11. DELICIOUS TURKEY WRAP

Total time: 20 minutes

Servings: 6

### Ingredients:

- 1 ¼ lb. ground turkey, lean
- 4 green onions, minced
- 1 tablespoon olive oil
- 1 garlic clove, minced
- 2 teaspoons chili paste
- 8 oz. water chestnuts, diced
- 3 tablespoons hoisin sauce
- 2 tablespoons coconut amino
- 1 tablespoon rice vinegar
- 12 butter lettuce leaves
- ⅛ teaspoon salt

### Directions:

1. Take a pan and place it over medium heat, add oil, turkey, and garlic to the pan.
2. Heat for 6 minutes until cooked.
3. Take a bowl and transfer turkey to the bowl.
4. Add onions and water chestnuts.

5. Stir in hoisin sauce, coconut amino, vinegar, salt, and chili paste.
6. Toss well and transfer the mix to lettuce leaves. Serve and enjoy.

Per serving: 162g calories, 4g fat, 7g carbs, 23g protein.

## 12. BACON AND CHICKEN GARLIC WRAP

Total time: 25 minutes

Servings: 4

**Ingredients:**

- 1 chicken fillet, cut into small cubes
- 8–9 thin slices bacon, cut to fit cubes
- 6 garlic cloves, minced

**Directions:**

1. Preheat your oven to 400° (F). Line a baking tray with aluminum foil.
2. Add minced garlic to a bowl and rub each chicken piece with it.
3. Wrap each garlic chicken bite in a slice of bacon and secure with a toothpick.

4. Transfer bites to the baking sheet, keeping a little bit of space between them.
5. Bake for about 15 to 20 minutes until crispy. Serve and enjoy.

Per serving: 260g calories, 19g fat, 5g carbs, 22g protein.

## 13. PUMPKIN PANCAKES

Total time: 25 minutes

Servings: 6

**Ingredients:**

- 3 large eggs, separate the egg whites for use
- ⅔ cup organic oats
- 6 oz. pumpkin puree
- 1 tablespoon collagen peptides
- 1 teaspoon stevia powder
- ½ teaspoon cinnamon
- Cooking spray

**Directions:**

1. Blend all the ingredients together to a smooth mixture.
2. Apply the cooking spray to the pan to coat and pour a

part of the batter into the pan and let it coat the pan properly.
3. Wait till the edges of the pancake brown up a little bit, then flip and cook from the other side.
4. Serve with fresh fruit.

Per serving: 70g calories, 16g carbs, 3g fat, 3g protein.

## 14. CHEDDAR HAM FRITTATA

Total time: 15 minutes

Servings: 2

**Ingredients:**

- 1 ⅔ cup ham, chopped
- 1 tablespoon shredded cheddar cheese
- 80g. spinach
- ⅔ cup chestnut mushrooms, diced
- 4 medium eggs
- 1 teaspoon oil

**Directions:**

1. Set the grill to its highest setting and leave it to heat up. Subsequently, in an ovenproof frying pan, heat the oil over a medium flame.

2. Fry the mushrooms in the pan for 2 minutes or until they soften. Add in the spinach and the ham and keep stirring them 1 minute longer after the spinach has wilted.
3. Spice with a pinch of salt and black pepper after the vegetables are cooked.
4. Lower the flame to pour in the beaten eggs and let them evenly spread and cook uninterrupted for 3 minutes–just enough time to let them set.
5. Put the cooked meal under the grill for 2 minutes after spritzing it with cheese. You can either serve it hot or cold, your choice.

Per serving: 226 calories, 22g protein, 15g fat, 1g fiber.

## 15. ORANGE RASP FRENCH TOAST

Total time: 10 minutes

Servings: 2

**Ingredients:**

- 2 tablespoons orange juice
- 2 medium eggs
- 2 slices spelt bread, halved
- 1 teaspoon rapeseed oil
- 1 ⅔ cups raspberries and blueberries

- Honey for serving

## Directions:

1. In a wide bowl, beat the orange juice and the eggs. Then, soak both sides of the bread in the mixture for about 2 minutes.
2. Put a non-stick frying pan over a high flame and drizzle the rapeseed oil on it.
3. When the pan is heated, cook the soaked bread for a few minutes without flipping it or it might break. Flip and cook the other side of the bread for 1 to 2 minutes.
4. Top the finished French toast with the berries and the honey.

Per serving: 197 calories, 10g fat, 14g protein, 10g carbs, 2g fiber.

## 16. CINNAMON STEVIA OATMEAL

Total time: 20 minutes

Servings: 1

### Ingredients:

- ¼ teaspoon cinnamon
- ½ cup old-fashioned Oats

- 1 cup unsweetened almond milk
- 2 packets Stevia or any other no-calorie sweetener
- 2 pinches salt

## Directions:

1. Switch on the stove and mix all the ingredients in a non-stick pot.
2. Pour in 1 cup of water and combine well.
3. Let the mixture boil and then reduce the flame down to a simmer. The gentle bubbling will cook the oats.
4. Continually keep stirring it until it's creamy and thick. When cooked, serve with blueberries and walnuts.

Per serving: 106g calories, 11.6g carbs, 3.8g fat, 3.3g fiber, 3.7g protein.

## LUNCH RECIPES

### 1. CHICKEN FARRO BOWL

Total time: 40 minutes

Servings: 4

**Ingredients:**

- 1 cup Bob's Red Mill farro, cooked
- 3 quarts water (or stock)
- ½ teaspoon salt
- 2 chicken breasts, boneless and skinless (1 pound)
- 3 tablespoons extra virgin olive oil
- 1 lemon zest
- 1 lemon, juiced
- 2 garlic cloves, grated

- 1 teaspoon dried oregano
- ¼ teaspoon black pepper
- 1 pint cherry tomatoes, halved
- 2 cups cucumbers, chopped
- 1 cup kalamata olives, pitted and sliced
- ½ red onion, chopped
- ½ cup feta cheese, crumbled
- Lemon wedges for serving
- Fresh dill and parsley for garnish
- 1 cup yogurt (plain)
- ¼ teaspoon dried dill

## Directions:

### For the bowls,

1. Rinse and drain the farro before using. Combine the farro, salt, and just enough water or stock to cover it in a saucepan. Bring to a boil, then simmer for 30 minutes over medium-low heat. Empty any accumulated water.
2. In a gallon zip bag, add the chicken breasts, olive oil, lemon zest, lemon juice, garlic, oregano, salt, and pepper. Marinate in the refrigerator for 4 hours or overnight.
3. In a large skillet over medium-high heat, heat the olive oil, then add the chicken breasts and cook for 7 minutes, flipping halfway through, or until they reach

an internal temperature of 165 degrees. Remove the marinade and throw it away.
4. Remove the chicken from the pan and set it aside to cool for 5 minutes before slicing.
5. To make the Greek bowls, start by putting a bed of farro in the bottom of your bowl or meal prep dish. Tzatziki sauce, feta cheese, tomatoes, cucumber, olives, red onion, and tzatziki sauce are served with sliced chicken. Serve with lemon wedges and a parsley and dill garnish.

**For the tzatziki sauce,**

1. Using a mesh sieve, line a big bowl, and in the sieve, lay a paper towel.
2. Grate the cucumber and garlic clove on a cheese grater, then drain to remove any extra liquid.
3. In a medium mixing bowl, combine the garlic, shredded cucumber, salt, yogurt, lemon juice, and dill. Chill for an hour before serving.

Per serving: 585 calories, 4.1g sugar, 1106.3mg sodium, 30.4g fat, 45.5g carbs, 8.8g fiber, 35.9g protein, 99.4g cholesterol.

## 2. SHRIMP FRIED RICE

Total time: 20 minutes

Servings: 4

**Ingredients:**

- 6 cups cauliflower rice, or 1 large head cauliflower
- ¼ cup tamari sauce, soy sauce, or coconut aminos
- 1 teaspoon honey
- ½ teaspoon ground ginger, or ½ teaspoon shredded fresh ginger
- 1 tablespoon crushed red pepper
- 1 tablespoon sesame seed oil
- 1 handful green onions, chopped (whites and greens separated)
- ½ cup frozen peas
- ½ cup carrots, diced
- 3 eggs, beaten
- ½ pound thawed, peeled, and deveined shrimp

**Directions:**

1. Chop cauliflower into bits and place in a food processor. After pulsing, set aside to finely chop until the mixture resembles rice.

2. Set aside a small bowl and combine the sauce of your choice, honey, ginger, and red pepper flakes.
3. In a large skillet or wok, heat sesame oil over medium-high heat. Add white potions of green onions and sauté for about a minute. Stir in the frozen peas and carrots and boil through for about 2 minutes. Place the vegetables on one side of the wok and add the beaten eggs to the other. Cook eggs on one side of the pan until done, moving the mixture around as it cooks. Cook for about 2 minutes, or until the shrimp have gone pink.
4. Stir in the riced cauliflower until everything is well combined. Pour the Tamari sauce mixture over the top, ensuring sure it is well distributed, and simmer for another 4 minutes, or until the cauliflower has softened but is still firm. Turn off the heat, add the green onions, and cover for a minute to soften.

Per serving: 205 calories, 5.7g sugar, 617g sodium, 7.9g fat, 14.3g carbs, 4.5g fiber, 21.4g protein, 230.7g cholesterol.

## 3. GRASS-FED BURGERS

Grass-fed liver burgers are one of my favourite weekday lunch options, and they're super easy to prepare ahead of time to enjoy throughout the week. This can be served over a bed of dark leafy greens with a simple homemade dressing for a B vitamin-rich lunch that promotes healthy methylation and detox pathways.

Total time: 20 minutes

Servings: 2

**Ingredients:**

- ½ pound ground grass-fed beef liver
- ½ pound grass-fed ground beef
- ¼ teaspoon garlic powder
- ½ tablespoon cumin powder
- Salt and pepper, to taste
- Cooking oil of choice

**Directions:**

1. In a mixing bowl, combine the ingredients and shape into patties.
2. On medium-high heat, heat the frying oil in a skillet.
3. Cook burgers in a skillet until done to your liking.
4. Refrigerate in an airtight container for up to 4 days.

Per serving: 423 calories, 19.5 fat, 32g protein, 28g carbs, 2g fiber, 80mg cholesterol, 4mg iron, 682mg sodium, 183mg calcium, 8g sugar.

## 4. SHRIMP AND AVOCADO SALAD

Total time: 10 minutes

Servings: 4

This salad is light and refreshing, and it only takes a few minutes to prepare. You can't ask for a healthier lunch than this one, which features delectable shrimp and creamy avocado. With the simplest seafood sauce you'll ever make on top, it's absolute bliss. Enjoy this Whole 30-compliant salad with shrimp, avocado, and a heart-healthy fat-based dressing.

**Ingredients:**

- 1 lb. shrimp, boiled and skinned
- 2 small gem lettuces
- 1 large avocado
- 1 tablespoon cilantro, chopped (or coriander)
- 1 teaspoon lemon juice
- Salt and pepper, to taste
- ½ cup mayonnaise
- 2 tablespoons sugar-free ketchup
- 1 teaspoon Worcestershire sauce, or 1 teaspoon coconut aminos
- A sprinkle of cayenne pepper, to taste

## Directions:

1. In a small mixing bowl, whisk together all of the sauce ingredients until smooth and well blended. Pour the mixture into a serving basin or a jug.
2. Using salt and pepper, season the shrimp. To keep the avocado from browning, peel and slice it, then throw it in lemon juice.
3. Tear the lettuce into bits and place on a serving platter or dish. Place the shrimp on top of the lettuce and nestle the avocado slices in between them. (Note: Divide the salad across four tiny single-serve salad dishes for optimal portion control.)
4. Garnish with a sprinkling of coriander (or cilantro). If desired, garnish with lemon slices. Refrigerate for up to 3 days in an airtight container.

Per serving: 3.9g carbs, 26.9g protein, 32.6g fat, calories 426.

### 5. BUFFALO CHICKEN CHOPPED SALAD

Total time: 25 minutes

Servings: 2

## Ingredients:

- 285g cooked chicken, diced

- 3 tablespoons butter, melted
- ¼ cup Franks red-hot sauce, or sriracha chili sauce
- 1 large head romaine lettuce, chopped
- 4 slices crisped bacon, crumbled
- 1 small carrot, sliced
- ¼ cup banana peppers or green bell peppers
- 4 green onions, finely sliced
- ½ cup cherry tomatoes, halved
- ¼ cup blue cheese crumbles
- 1 large avocado, chopped
- 6 tablespoons ranch dressing

**Directions:**

1. Toss the chicken with the melted butter and buffalo sauce in a medium mixing bowl.
2. Combine the dressing ingredients in a small container.
3. Divide the salad ingredients among three salad dishes, then top with the chicken and drizzle with the dressing.
4. Serve right away or keep refrigerated for up to 2 days.

Per serving: 8.7g carbs, 42.2g protein, 46.4g fat, and 642 calories.

## 6. SALMON SESAME PAK CHOI

Total time: 20 minutes

Servings: 2

**Ingredients:**

- 2 skinless salmon fillets
- 1 tablespoon sweet chili sauce
- 1 tablespoon sesame seed oil
- 1 tablespoon dry sherry or mirin
- 2 teaspoons soy sauce
- 2 tablespoons ginger, finely grated
- brown rice or noodles (optional, to serve)
- 2 big pak choi
- 2 tablespoons vegetable oil
- 3 garlic cloves, grated
- ⅓ cup stock (fish or veggie)
- 2 teaspoons sesame seeds, toasted, for sprinkling

**Directions:**

1. Preheat the oven to 350 degrees (F) and in a shallow baking dish, place the fish. In a small dish, combine the honey, soy and sesame oil, mirin, sweet chilli, and ginger; pour over the salmon steaks until completely covered. Bake for 10 minutes.

2. To separate the leaves, cut a slice across the base of the pak choi. In a wok, heat the oils, then add the garlic and stir-fry for a few minutes to soften it. Fry the pak choi leaves until they begin to wilt. Pour in the stock, cover the pan tightly, and cook for 5 minutes—you want the pak choi stems to be soft but still have a bite to them.
3. Serve the pak choi with the salmon steaks in shallow dishes on top and the liquids spooned over the top. Serve on its own or with brown rice or noodles, strewn with toasted sesame seeds.

Per serving: 517 calories, 30g fat, 17g carbs, 15g sugar, 3g fiber, 4g protein, 2.8g salt.

## 7. GRILLED CHICKEN SALAD

Total time: 30 minutes

Serving: 4

### Ingredients:

- 2 boneless, skinless chicken breasts
- 1 teaspoon coriander powder
- 1 teaspoon dried oregano
- salt and pepper
- 5 tablespoons extra-virgin olive oil

- 4 tablespoons red wine vinegar
- 1 tablespoon parsley, freshly chopped
- 4 romaine hearts, chopped
- 3 Persian cucumbers, finely sliced
- 1 cup grape or cherry tomatoes, halved
- 2 avocados, sliced
- 4 oz. crumbled feta
- ½ cup kalamata olives, pitted and halved

**Directions:**

1. Preheat the grill to medium-high heat. Season the chicken with the coriander, oregano, salt, and pepper. Cook the chicken for 18 to 22 minutes, until golden and no longer pink, flipping halfway through. Allow chicken to rest for 5 minutes before slicing.
2. Prepare the dressing in the meantime. In a small bowl, combine the red wine vinegar, olive oil, and parsley; season with salt and pepper.
3. Filled four serving dishes with tomatoes, avocado, lettuce, cucumbers, feta, and olives. Drizzle the dressing over the cut chicken.

Per serving: 17g fat, 113g cholesterol, 517mg sodium, 705mg potassium, 7.6g carbs, 2.2g fiber.

## 8. STEAK FAJITA POWER BOWL

Total time: 45 minutes

Servings: 4

**Ingredients:**

- 2 tablespoons vegetable oil
- ½ yellow onion, half-moons cut
- 2 bell peppers, finely sliced
- salt and pepper
- 1 pound skirt steak, thinly sliced
- lime juice from half a lime
- 1 tablespoon cumin
- ½ teaspoon chili powder
- 4 cups brown rice, cooked
- 1 cup drained and rinsed black beans
- 1 cup frozen corn, warmed
- 1 avocado, finely sliced
- 1 tablespoon cilantro, coarsely chopped (to garnish)
- Sour cream (to serve)

**Directions:**

1. Heat 1 tablespoon vegetable oil in a large skillet over medium heat. Add the onions and peppers and season with salt and pepper to taste. Cook for 7 to 10 minutes,

or until onions are transparent and peppers are soft. Remove the skillet from the heat and set aside.
2. Allow the remaining vegetable oil to heat for about 30 seconds before adding the skirt steak to the pan. Squeeze half a lime over the steak and then season with chili powder, salt, cumin, and pepper. Allow it to cook for a minute or two to acquire a beautiful sear, then cook till done to your liking, roughly 5 minutes for an average well-done steak. Take pan away from the heat.
3. Build bowls: 1 cup rice in each bowl is a good starting point. Onions, steak, peppers, black beans, avocado, and corn go on top.
4. Serve with a sour cream drizzle and cilantro garnish.

Per serving: 390 calories, 11g fat, 1630g sodium, 47g carbs, 4g fiber, 6g glucose, 23g protein.

## 9. MANGO CHILI CHICKEN STIR-FRY

Total time: 30 minutes

Servings: 4

### Ingredients:

- ½ tablespoons sesame oil
- 1 tablespoon low-sodium soy sauce
- 1 tablespoon cornstarch

- 1 lb. boneless, skinless chicken thighs, diced
- ½ tablespoon peanut oil
- 1 tablespoon fresh ginger, minced
- 1 red onion, chopped
- 2 cups snow peas
- 1 tablespoon chili garlic sauce
- 1 mango, peeled and chopped
- ⅛ teaspoon sea salt
- ⅛ teaspoon black pepper

**Directions:**

1. In a large mixing bowl, combine sesame oil, soy sauce, cornstarch, and chicken; let sit for at least 20 minutes.
2. In a large skillet, heat peanut oil and then sauce, ginger, and onion for about 2 minutes; add snow peas and stir-fry for about 1 minute. Add chicken with the marinade and stir-fry for about 2 minutes or until chicken is browned. Add chili sauce, mango, salt, and pepper, and continue stir-frying for 1 minute or until chicken is cooked through and mango is tender. Serve over cooked brown rice.

Per serving: 354 calories, 12.4g fat, 23.8g carbs, 4.3g fiber, 36.8 protein.

## 10. TURKEY WITH CAPERS, TOMATOES, AND GREEN BEANS

Total time: 35 minutes

Servings: 4

**Ingredients:**

- 1 tablespoon extra-virgin olive oil
- 6 oz. turkey
- ¼ cup capers
- ¼ cup fresh tomatoes, diced
- Steamed green beans (to serve)

**Directions:**

1. Heat oil in a pan; add turkey and fry until golden brown and cooked through.
2. Remove the cooked turkey from the pan and transfer to a plate; add capers and tomatoes to the pan and cook until juicy. Spoon the caper mixture over the turkey and serve with steamed green beans.

Per serving: 111 calories, 5.7g fat, 1.8g carbs, 0.9g fiber, 5.7g protein.

## 11. THAI FISH CURRY

Total time: 15 minutes

Servings: 6

**Ingredients:**

- 1 ⅓ cup olive oil
- 1 ½ lb. salmon fillets
- 2 cups coconut milk, freshly squeezed
- 2 tablespoons curry powder
- 1 ¼ cup cilantro, chopped
- Salt and pepper, to taste

**Directions:**

1. In your instant pot, add in all ingredients. Apply a seasoning of salt and pepper. Give a good stir.
2. Set the lid in place and the vent to point to "Sealing."
3. Set the instant pot to "Manual" and cook for 10 minutes.
4. Do a quick pressure release.

Per serving: 470 calories, 5.6g carbs, and 25.5g protein.

## 12. FRIED TOFU WITH TENDER SPRING GREENS

Total time: 35 minutes

Servings: 3

### Ingredients:

- 2 tablespoons extra-virgin olive oil
- 14 oz. extra-firm tofu, sliced
- 1 medium onion, thinly sliced
- 1 medium yellow or red bell pepper, chopped
- 2 teaspoons fresh ginger, grated
- 12 oz. spring greens, chopped
- 3 tablespoons teriyaki sauce
- ¼ cup toasted cashews, chopped

### Directions:

1. Add half oil to a pan and set over medium heat. Add tofu and fry until golden. Transfer to a plate.
2. Add the remaining oil to the pan and sauté onion until translucent. Stir in bell pepper and continue sautéing until the onion is tender and golden. Stir in ginger and greens until wilted.
3. Stir in tofu and season with teriyaki sauce. Top with toasted cashews to serve.

Per serving: 338 calories, 22.7g fat, 20.8g carbs, 6.9g fiber, 19.3g protein.

## 13. SATISFYING TURKEY LETTUCE WRAPS

Total time: 35 minutes

Servings: 4

### Ingredients:

- ½ lb. ground turkey
- ½ small onion, finely chopped
- 1 garlic clove, minced
- 2 tablespoons extra-virgin olive oil
- 1 head lettuce
- 1 teaspoon cumin
- ½ tablespoon fresh ginger, sliced
- 2 tablespoons apple cider vinegar
- 2 tablespoons cilantro, freshly chopped
- 1 teaspoon black pepper
- 1 teaspoon sea salt

### Directions:

1. Sauté garlic and onion in olive oil until fragrant and translucent.
2. Add turkey and cook well.

3. Stir in the remaining ingredients and continue cooking for 5 minutes more.
4. To serve, ladle a spoonful of turkey mixture onto a lettuce leaf and wrap.

Per serving: 192 calories, 13.6g fat, 4.6g carbs, 1g fiber, 16.3g protein.

# DINNER RECIPES

## 1. TURKEY TACOS

Total time: 25 minutes

Servings: 4

**Ingredients:**

- 2 teaspoons oil
- 1 little red onion, sliced
- 1 garlic clove, coarsely chopped
- 1 pound ground extra-lean turkey
- 1 tablespoon sodium-free taco seasoning
- 8 whole-grain corn tortillas, warmed
- ¼ cup sour cream
- ½ cup shredded Mexican cheese

- 1 avocado, sliced
- Salsa (to serve)
- 1 cup lettuce, chopped

## Directions:

1. Heat the oil in a large skillet over medium-high heat. Cook, turning occasionally, until the onion is soft, about 5 to 6 minutes. Cook for 1 minute after adding the garlic.
2. Cook, breaking up the turkey with a spoon until it is nearly brown, about 5 minutes. Add 1 cup water and taco seasoning. Cook for 7 minutes, or until the liquid has been reduced by little more than half.
3. To serve, stuff the turkey-filled tortillas with cheese, sour cream, salsa, avocado, and lettuce.

Per serving: 28g protein, 27g fat, 30g carbs, 47 calories.

### 2. SPAGHETTI BOLOGNESE

Total time: 1 hour 30 minutes

Servings: 4

## Ingredients:

- 1 large spaghetti squash
- 3 tablespoons olive oil
- ½ tablespoon garlic powder
- salt and pepper
- 1 onion, finely chopped
- 1 ¼ lb. ground turkey
- 4 garlic cloves, finely chopped
- 8 oz. tiny cremini mushrooms, cut into pieces
- 3 cups fresh tomatoes, chopped (or two 15 oz. cans)
- 1 8 oz. can low-sodium, sugar-free tomato sauce
- basil leaves, chopped

## Directions:

1. Preheat the oven to 400 degrees (F). Remove the seeds from the spaghetti squash and cut it in half lengthwise. Each half should be rubbed with 1/2 tbsp. oil and seasoned with garlic powder, salt, and pepper. Roast until soft, 35 to 40 minutes, skin-side up on a rimmed baking sheet. Allow 10 minutes for cooling.
2. Meanwhile, heat the remaining 2 tablespoons of oil in a large skillet over medium heat. Cook, turning periodically, for 6 minutes, until the onion is soft, seasoning with salt and pepper. Cook, breaking up the turkey into small pieces with a spoon, until browned,

about 6 to 7 minutes. Add garlic and cook for 1 minute.
3. Place the turkey on one side of the pan and the mushrooms on the other. Cook for 5 minutes, stirring periodically, until the mushrooms are cooked. Combine with the turkey. Add tomatoes and tomato sauce and simmer for 10 minutes.
4. Scoop out the squash and place it on plates while the sauce simmers. Serve with a dollop of turkey bolognese and a sprinkling of basil, if desired.

Each serving: 450 calories, 32g protein, 31g carbs, 6g fiber, 23g fat.

## 3. CHICKEN WITH FRIED CAULIFLOWER RICE

Total time: 35 minutes

Servings: 4

**Ingredients:**

- 2 tablespoons grapeseed oil
- 1 ¼ pound boneless, skinless chicken breast, pounded to a uniform thickness
- 4 big eggs, beaten
- 2 red bell peppers, finely sliced
- 2 carrots, finely sliced

- 1 onion, finely chopped
- 2 garlic cloves, finely chopped
- ½ cup frozen peas, thawed
- 4 cups cauliflower rice
- 2 tablespoons low-sodium soy sauce
- 2 tablespoons rice vinegar
- salt and pepper

**Directions:**

1. Heat 1 tbsp. oil over medium-high heat in a large, deep skillet. Cook chicken for 3 to 4 minutes per side, or until golden brown on both sides. Transfer to a cutting board and let cool for 6 minutes before slicing. Add the remaining 1 tbsp. oil to the same skillet. Scramble the eggs for 1 to 2 minutes, or until they are just set; transfer to a bowl.
2. Cook the bell pepper, carrot, and onion until barely tender, stirring regularly, about 4 to 5 minutes. Add the garlic and cook for 1 minute. Toss with peas and scallions before serving.
3. Combine the cauliflower, soy sauce, rice vinegar, salt, and pepper in a mixing bowl. Allow the cauliflower to sit for 2 to 3 minutes, stirring occasionally, until it starts to turn color. In a mixing bowl, combine the sliced chicken and eggs.

Per serving: 427 calories, 45g protein, 25g carbs, 7g fiber, 16g fat.

## 4. SHEET-PAN STEAK

Total time: 50 minutes

Servings: 4

**Ingredients:**

- 1 pound cremini mushrooms, trimmed and halved
- ¼ pound broccoli, trimmed and cut into 2-inch lengths
- 4 garlic cloves, finely chopped
- 3 tablespoons olive oil
- ¼ teaspoon red pepper flakes (or more to taste)
- salt and pepper
- 2 1-inch thick New York strip steaks, trimmed of extra fat
- 1 15 oz. can low-sodium cannellini beans, washed

**Directions:**

1. Preheat the oven to 450 degrees (F). Toss the broccoli, mushrooms, red pepper flakes, garlic, oil, salt, and pepper on a wide rimmed baking sheet. Bake for 15 minutes.
2. To make room for the steaks, push the mixture to the

pan's edges. Place the steaks in the center of the pan and season with 1/4 tsp. salt and pepper. Roast the steaks until they're done to your liking, about 5 to 7 minutes on each side for medium-rare. Allow 5 minutes for the steaks to rest on a cutting board before slicing.
3. Toss the beans with the rest of the ingredients on the baking sheet. Roast for 3 minutes, or until thoroughly heated. Serve steak with beans and veggies.

Per serving: 464 calories, 42g protein, 26g carbs, 8g fiber, 22g fat.

## 5. ZOODLES WITH KETO ALFREDO SAUCE

Total time: 20 minutes

Servings: 2

**Ingredients:**

- 1 cup cashews, unsalted, soaked and raw, or 1 ½ cup cauliflower, cooked
- Half teacup bone broth prepared from chicken bones
- 3 tablespoons Bulletproof grass-fed ghee, and additional for frying
- 2 tablespoons Bulletproof Unflavoured Collagen Powder

- ¾ teaspoon mustard powder
- ¾ teaspoon garlic powder
- ¼–½ tablespoon onion powder
- salt, to taste
- 2 diced brown onions
- 4–5 strips of bacon, chopped
- Two servings of zoodles
- 2 garlic cloves, smashed

**Directions:**

1. In a blender, combine bone broth, ghee, and soaked (and filtered) cashews or cooked cauliflower (or butter), onion, garlic, collagen powder, and mustard powder. Blitz until smooth. Taste. Then season with salt to flavor.
2. In ghee, fry onions till golden brown. Add the bacon to the pan and cook until it begins to crisp up. Stir in the garlic. Remove from heat once all ingredients are golden brown and bacon is crispy.
3. In a medium pot, steam zoodles until they are cooked to your taste.
4. Meanwhile, reheat the alfredo sauce in another small pot over medium heat.
5. Divide the cooked zoodles between two plates. Serve with crispy bacon and onions on top of the sauce. If

preferred, top with fresh herbs and a pinch of salt and pepper.

Per serving: 765 calories, 62g fat, 105mg cholesterol, 1071mg salt, 31g carbs, 9g fibre, 15.3g sugar, 26g protein.

## 6. PORK TENDERLOIN WITH BUTTERNUT SQUASH AND BRUSSELS SPROUTS

Total time: 50 minutes

Servings: 4

**Ingredients:**

- 1 ¾ pound pork tenderloin, trimmed
- Salt and pepper, to taste
- 3 tablespoons canola oil
- 2 fresh thyme sprigs
- 2 garlic cloves, peeled
- 4 cups Brussels sprouts, trimmed and halved
- 4 cups butternut squash, chopped

## Directions:

1. Preheat oven to 400 degrees (F). Season the tenderloin with salt and pepper. Heat 1 tbsp. oil in a big cast-iron pan over medium high heat. When the oil begins to shimmer, add the tenderloin and sear for 8 to 12 minutes, or until golden brown on all sides. Place on a plate to cool.
2. Add the thyme and garlic to the pan with the remaining 2 tbsp. oil and heat for 1 minute, or until fragrant. Combine the Brussels sprouts, butternut squash, and a generous amount of salt and pepper in a large mixing bowl. Cook, stirring occasionally, for 4 to 6 minutes, or until the veggies are slightly browned.
3. Place the tenderloin on top of the vegetables and roast for 15 to 20 minutes, or until the veggies are soft and the tenderloin reaches an internal temperature of 140°.
4. Carefully remove the skillet from the oven while using oven mitts. Allow for 5 minutes of resting time before slicing and serving the tenderloin with the vegetables. To serve as a side, toss greens with a balsamic vinaigrette.

Per serving: 401 calories, 44g protein, 25g carbs, 6g fiber, 15g fats.

## 7. BEEF AND CARROT STEW

Total time: 70 minutes

Servings: 6

**Ingredients:**

- 1½ pounds beef stew meat, trimmed and chopped
- 4 cups beef broth
- 1 tablespoon olive oil
- Salt and pepper, to taste
- 2 garlic cloves, minced
- 1 cup tomato puree
- 1 teaspoon dried parsley
- 1 teaspoon dried rosemary
- 3 carrots, peeled and sliced
- 1 teaspoon onion powder
- ½ tablespoon dried thyme
- 1 tablespoon paprika
- 3 tablespoons fresh parsley, chopped
- 1 teaspoon garlic powder

**Instructions:**

1. Combine the beef cubes, salt, and pepper in a large mixing bowl and toss well to coat.

2. Heat the oil in a Dutch oven over medium-high heat and brown the meat cubes for around 4–5 minutes.
3. Stir in the other ingredients until well combined.
4. Turn the heat up to high and bring the mixture to a boil, then reduce the heat to low and continue to cook, covered, for another 40–50 minutes.
5. Remove from the heat and stir in the salt and pepper. Serve immediately.

Per serving: 295 calories, 10.5g fat, 644mg sodium, 8g carbs, 2.2g fiber, 4g sugar, 39g protein.

# CONCLUSION

Fasting was once associated with religious or philosophical rituals and practices. However, depending on their goals and circumstances, an increasing number of fitness enthusiasts are beginning to adopt intermittent fasting into their lives as a strategy to lose weight, improve physical health, and extend their lives.

Intermittent fasting makes perfect sense from an evolutionary standpoint. On a daily basis, our palaeolithic forebears had either plenty of meat or a scarcity of it. As a result, during periods of nutritional restriction, we progressed.

When resources are scarce, the body switches on "repair and care" genes. These genes help to promote the production of important molecules like glutathione, which aids in the repair of tissues that would otherwise go unrepaired during periods of abundance. As a result of this adaptation, cells will live longer.

The diet pattern that includes a period of fasting followed by a period of eating is referred to as intermittent fasting. It can be done in a number of different ways. A feast day frequently precedes an alternate-day fast, in which you eat as much as you want one day and then fast the next. On a less regimented schedule, a single twenty-four-hour fast can be completed once a week, once a month, or whenever you like. You may skip a meal on a regular or irregular basis.

The simplified eating window is the method I recommend. It entails cramming the equivalent of a full day's worth of food into a set number of hours. Someone might, for example, eat from 7:00 a.m. until 3:00 p.m. The next day, they'll take it easy before 7 a.m. As a result, their body would take a sixteen-hour break from digestion. And that happens from time to time, without much consideration.

When people hear the word "fasting," they frequently conjure up images of starvation. People become jittery as a result of not eating every few hours. What would happen if their metabolism suddenly ceased to function? Aren't they all going to die at the same time? Isn't it true that if they resume feeding, everything will be processed as fat?

It's not about punishing oneself when fasting on a regular basis. It's as simple as fasting for a short period of time and then returning to your normal routine. Eating like a rabbit all of the time is a surefire way to lose weight and manipulate your diet. By eating like a rabbit for the majority of the day and retaining balance and power, you can improve your weight-loss efforts and meet your goals.

In conclusion, none of the aforementioned worries should be a substantial source of concern. If a person's health is stable—that is, they have no underlying medical disease or illness, such as diabetes—skipping a meal or two can help them maintain a healthy lifestyle.

Almost every diet book you'll discover in a bookstore uses a tactic to persuade the reader to eat less. Calorie counting takes time and can be aggravating. Reading labels and weighing ingredients can quickly take away from the enjoyment of dinner preparation. It's difficult enough to follow a recipe, but having to make replacements or give up full parts of a meal to keep inside a calorie limit is not something most people want to do. As a result of such measures, the diet ends up totally abandoned.

Intermittent fasting is a more effective technique to lose weight or maintain weight. There are a few different ways to go about doing this. Brad Pilon, author of Eat Stop Eat, suggests fasting for a complete twenty-four hours. It's not a bad technique because you'll significantly reduce your calorie consumption if you don't go overboard. The disadvantage is that going a whole day without meals is a psychological hurdle that some individuals might find difficult to conquer.

Others advise packing their entire days' worth of calories into a four- to nine-hour period of time. This, too, is dependent on calorie counting and diet adherence. To avoid having to worry about what to eat when it's time to eat, plan your meals a few days ahead of time. Simply cook the prepared dishes and go about your business.

While all of these strategies are effective and serve their purposes, a more relaxed approach can also be a good place to start. Many folks will be perfectly fine to skip breakfast, eat a late lunch, and a light early dinner. Drinking enough water during the fasting period will assist to keep hunger at bay.

Depending on the quantity of the meals you're eating, skipping a meal or two between three and five times each week can help you lose between 1500 and 2500 calories. When you sum it all up, you're looking at a weekly net calorie loss of around a pound. A smaller deficit can be troublesome because it will take you longer to reach your goals. A larger deficit, on the other hand, is easier to manage. A diet that you can stick to is ideal.

Finally, it makes no difference whether you skip an entire day's worth of meals, eat one meal at a time, or monitor calories and fit them into an "eating slot." The calorie reduction that results will help you lose weight while also improving your health and well-being.

This book takes you on a road to a healthier lifestyle. It has demonstrated how many elements affect one's well-being and health. Its purpose is to inform you of the numerous options available to you. Remember all of the options I've presented to you, including diet alternatives and specific food sources that can trigger autophagy in the brain.

It is now your responsibility to decide which of these food sources or improvements will work for you, and remember to experiment, noting which ones make you feel great and which ones you prefer to avoid. With all of this information, you can decide which options best suit your lifestyle and preferences. As you carry all of this information forward, it may seem overwhelming to begin applying it to your own life. Keep in mind that life is a cycle, and you shouldn't expect perfection from yourself. You are already changing your life by reading this book.

# DOWNLOAD YOUR FREE CHEAT SHEET

*(Don't start fasting before you've consulted this cheat sheet...)*

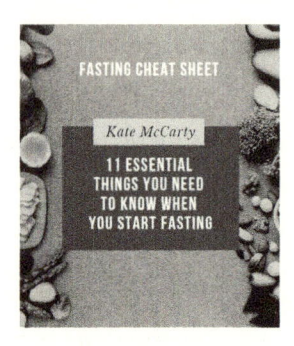

This cheat sheet includes:

- 11 things to know and to do while you are fasting.
- Why you need to know those things to start successfully.
- These things will make the process easier and more enjoyable.

The last thing I want is that the fasting process will be uncomfortable.

To receive your fasting cheat sheet, scan this QR code:

# REFERENCES

"7 Do's and Don'ts for Intermittent Fasting." iSatori [Blog]. n.d. https://www.isatori.com/blogs/articles/intermittent-fasting-dos-donts.

"A Woman's Changing Body." CanyonRanch [Blog]. n.d. https://www.canyonranch.com/blog/health/a-womans-changing-body/.

Bjarnadottir, A. "Beginner's Guide to the 5:2 Diet." *Healthline*. May 31, 2018. https://www.healthline.com/nutrition/the-5-2-diet-guide#TOC_TITLE_HDR_7.

Bohn, P. *Intermittent Fasting After 50*. 2020.

Buice, D. "7 Healthy Habits for a Healthy Life." *Living Magazine*. n.d. https://www.google.com/amp/s/www.livingmagazine.net/7-healthy-habits-healthy-life/amp/.

# REFERENCES

Butler, N. "How To Begin Intermittent Fasting." *Medical News Today*. April 4, 2019. https://www.medicalnewstoday.com/articles/324882#summary.

Calfuray, S. *Intermittent Fasting for Women Over 50, An In-Depth Guide with Explanations, Exercises, Recipes and Much More*. 2021.

Fletcher, J. "How To Begin Intermittent Fasting." *National Institute of Health*. April 4, 2019. https://www.diddk.nih.gov/health-information/diet-nutritional/changes-habits-better-health.

Gunnars, K. "10 Evidence-Based Health Benefits of Intermittent Fasting." *Healthline*. May 13, 2021. https://www.healthline.com/nutrition/10-health-benefits-of-intermittent-fasting#TOC_TITLE_HDR_11.

Gunnars, K. "Intermittent Fasting 101—The Ultimate Beginner's Guide." *Healthline*. April 20, 2020. https://www.healthline.com/nutrition/intermittent-fasting-guide#what-it-is.

Hill, A. (2020, January 7) "Eat Stop Eat Review: Does It Work for Weight Loss?" January 7, 2020. https://www.healthline.com/nutrition/eat-stop-eat-review#effectivess.

"How To Prepare Yourself Before Starting Intermittent Fasting." *Meds News*. August 19, 2020. https://www.medsnews.com/health/preparing-before-intermittent-fasting/.

"Intermittent Fasting: What Is It, and How Does It Work?" Johns Hopkins Medicine. n.d. https://www.hopkinsmedicine. org/health/wellness-and-prevention-/intermittent-fasting-what-is-it-and-how-does-it-work.

Link, R. "What Are the Different Stages of Fasting?" *Healthline.* January 19, 2021. https://www.healthline.com/nutrition/stages-of-fasting#1,-fed-state.

Melone, L. "Body Changes After 50: How Much Can You Really Control?" Next Avenue. December 5, 2016. https://www.nextavenue.org/body-changes-50-control/.

"Need an Intermittent Fasting Meal Plan? Here's Your 7-Day Brunch and Dinner Plan To Break Your Fast." *Women's Health Magazine.* January 30, 2020. https://www.womenshealthmag.com/weight-loss/amp30658778/.

Oshin, M. (2018, July 2) "11 Lessons Learned from 4 Years of Intermittent Fasting: The Good and Bad." The Ladders. July 2, 2018, https://www.theladders.com/career-advice/11-lessons-learned-from-4-years-of-intermittent-fasting-the-good-and-bad.

Swiner, C. "What to Expect in Your 50s." WebMD: Compass [Website]. June 29, 2021. https://www.webmd.com/healthy-aging/ss/slideshow-what-to-expect-in-your-50s.

Van Hare, H., and Siefert, R. (2020, March 2) "Ways You Didn't Know Your Body Changes After 50." *The Daily Meal.* March 2,

2020. https://www.thedailymeal.com/healthy-eating/body-changes-after-50gallery.

Wilson, J. *Intermittent Fasting for Women Over 50*. 2021.

# References

1. Kris Gunnars. Intermittent fasting 101- the ultimate beginners guide.

https://www.healthline.com/nutrition/intermittent-fasting-guide#what-it-is

2. John Hopkins medicine.

https://www.hopkinsmedicine.org/health/wellness-and-prevention-/intermittent-fasting-what-is-it-and-how-does-it-work

3. Katherine Marengo LDN, R.D. 10 evidence based health benefits of intermittent fasting

https://www.healthline.com/nutrition/10-health-benefits-of-intermittent-fasting#TOC_TITLE_HDR_11

4. Rachel Link.MS.RD. "What are the different stages of fasting?"

https://www.healthline.com/nutrition/stages-of-fasting#1,-fed-state

5. Jennifer Wilson. (2021, June 15) "Intermittent fasting for women over 50"

6. Holly Van Hare and Rosie Siefert (2020, March 2) 'ways you didn't know your body changes after 50'

https://www.thedailymeal.com/healthy-eating/body-changes-after-50gallery

7. Carmelita Swiner, MD (2021, June 29) "what to expect in your 50s"

https://www.webmd.com/healthy-aging/ss/slideshow-what-to-expect-in-your-50s

8. Linda Melone, CSCS (2016, December 5) "body changes after 50: How much can you really control?"

https://www.nextavenue.org/body-changes-50-control/

9. Canyon Ranch. A Woman's changing body.

https://www.canyonranch.com/blog/health/a-womans-changing-body/

10. Adder Bjarnadottir (2018, may 31) beginners guide to the 5:2 diet

https://www.healthline.com/nutrition/the-5-2-diet-guide#TOC_TITLE_HDR_7

11. Ansley Hill (2020, January 7) eat stop eat review. Does it work for weight loss?

https://www.healthline.com/nutrition/eat-stop-eat-review#effectivess

12. Dos and don'ts for intermittent fasting

https://www.isatori.com/blogs/articles/intermittent-fasting-dos-donts

13. Mayo Oshin (2018, July 2) lessons learned from 4 year of intermittent fasting: the good and bad

https://www.theladders.com/career-advice/11-lessons-learned-from-4-years-of-intermittent- fasting-the - good-and-bad

14. Natalie Butler (2019, April 4th) how to begin intermittent fasting

https://www.medicalnewstoday.com/articles/324882#summary

15. Meds news-health and medicine information: how to prepare yourself before starting intermittent fasting.

# REFERENCES | 183

https://www.medsnews.com/health/preparing-before-intermittent-fasting/

16. Jenna fletcher (2019,April 4)how to begin intermittent fasting https://www.diddk.nih.gov/health-information/diet-nutritional/changes-habits-better-health

17. 7 healthy habits for a healthy life https://www.google.com/amp/s/www.livingmagazine.net/7-healthy-habits-healthy-life/amp/

18. Men's health guide to intermittent fasting.

https://www.womenshealthmag.com/weight-loss/amp30658778/

19. Patricia, Bohn. (2020, August 13) intermittent fasting after 50.

20. The Men's Health Guide to Intermittent Fasting: Build Muscle and Torch Fat without Stressing about What You Eat www.womenshealthmag.com/weight-loss/amp30658778/ intermittent-fasting-meal-plan-men-s-health/

21. Sayen Calfuray (2021,July 1) intermittent fasting for women over 50,an in-depth guide with explanations, exercises, recipes and much more to undertake the path of the intermittent fasting for women over 50

Made in the USA
Monee, IL
17 March 2022